Urinary
Incontinence in
Primary Care

Urinary Incontinence in Primary Care

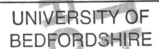
Linda Cardozo MD FRCOG
Professor of Urogynaecology, King's College Hospital, London, UK

David Staskin MD
Director, Urodynamics and Incontinence Center, Boston, USA

Michael Kirby MB BS LRCP MRCS MRCP
Family Practitioner, The Surgery, Letchworth, UK

with a contribution from
Angela Billington RGN RM DipHV
Clinical Nurse Specialist, Continence Advisory Service, Baldock, UK

I S I S
MEDICAL
M E D I A

British Library Cataloguing-in Publication Data.
A catalogue record for this title is available from
the British Library.

ISBN 1 901865 68 1

Cardozo, L. (Linda)
Urinary Incontinence in Primary Care
Linda Cardozo, David Staskin, Michael Kirby

Always refer to the manufacturer's Prescribing
Information before prescribing drugs cited in this book.

Typeset by
Creative Associates, Oxford

Image Reproduction
Acumen overseas PTE Ltd

Design
Ellen Moorcraft

Technical Editor
Christine Mckillop PhD

Isis Medical Media staff
Commissioning Editor: John Harrison
Editorial Controller: Fiona Cornell
Production Controller: Geoff Holdsworth

Printed and bound by
Craft Print International Ltd., Singapore

Distributed in the USA by
Books International, Inc., PO Box 605,
Herndon, VA 20172, USA

Distributed in the rest of the world by
Plymbridge Distributors Ltd., Estover Road,
Plymouth PL6 7PY, UK

CONTENTS

I OVERVIEW FROM THE PRIMARY CARE PERSPECTIVE

Urinary incontinence regularly disrupts the lives of about 5% of home-dwelling adults. It is a common problem at all ages but is most prevalent in the elderly, especially among those living in an institution. According to The Continence Foundation, one in four women and one in nine men will suffer from urinary incontinence at some stage of their lives.[1] The mortality rate from incontinence is low and it is clear that patients do not want to talk about it. A Gallup survey performed in 1994 showed that almost 70% of sufferers put up with their symptoms and failed to seek medical advice.[2] The majority of those who eventually seek help do so only after an average of four years of enduring the symptoms and unhappiness this condition causes. In the UK, unlike the US, Primary Care Groups (PCGs) have the responsibility for buying continence promotion, education and support services from community trusts and voluntary agencies. They are also responsible for establishing contracts to ensure that adequate supply networks exist for continence projects.

> One in four women and one in nine men will suffer from urinary incontinence at some stage of their lives.

ECONOMIC ISSUES

The costs of continence care are hard to calculate accurately because incontinence is grossly under reported by sufferers and undiagnosed by primary health care teams. In the UK, incontinence costs the National Health Service (NHS) an estimated £70 million a year in pads and aids alone.[3] In the USA, the use of continence pads costs US$ 1000 per person per year, as estimated by the US Consensus Conference on Incontinence.[4] On top of this must be added the cost to the individual in terms of impaired quality of life and the cost to the NHS of diagnosis and treatment. Yet, this common and costly

> In the UK, incontinence costs the National Health Service (NHS) an estimated £70 million a year in pads and aids alone. In the USA, the use of continence pads costs US$ 1000 per person per year.

problem is eminently treatable in the community setting. There is international support for the belief that, despite an initial increase in costs resulting from improvements in diagnosis, there should be a long-term decrease in the national cost of incontinence with such measures.

EDUCATION

Inadequate training has been a major obstacle to the improved management of urinary incontinence in primary care. One study demonstrated a lack of knowledge amongst general practitioners (GPs) about the different types of incontinence and their causes, assessment and treatment.[5] A survey conducted in the UK showed that only 3% of GPs regarded their training in the subject as completely adequate and 14% said they had received no guidance whatsoever on managing the problem.[6] The majority of GPs (62%) said that they gained what knowledge they had about urinary incontinence during their general medical training, while only 34% had received any postgraduate education and only 9% had any specialist knowledge in the subject.[6]

INCONTINENCE MANAGEMENT

History taking by the primary health care team can be time consuming, examination may be embarrassing and for many primary care physicians, the temptation to refer to a specialist may be overwhelming. The success of any planned programme to improve the management of this condition will depend on the effectiveness of the patient's initial contact with the primary health care team. What is required is a short history to distinguish genuine stress incontinence (GSI) from detrusor instability or voiding difficulties, in combination with an examination which should cover the following aspects:

A short history to distinguish genuine stress incontinence (GSI) from detrusor instability or voiding difficulties is required in combination with an examination on the abdomen, the perineal area plus a digital rectal examination in men and a vaginal examination in women.

- The abdomen to detect masses, supra-pubic fullness or tenderness and, if possible, a post-void residual estimation
- The perineal area to assess the condition of the skin, which may be sore from persistent wetness, to check for genital atrophy, prolapse and pelvic mass, and to assess the pelvic floor tone
- Vaginal foreign bodies and infection also need to be excluded

- In men, in addition to the abdominal examination, a digital rectal examination should be performed to assess the prostate gland.

If indicated, a general physical examination should follow, looking for oedema, any neurological abnormality especially of the S_2–S_4 segments, general mobility, manual dexterity and mental state. A sample of urine should be sent for culture and sensitivities and, if there is haematuria, for cytology. Other assessments that are helpful include a voiding record and environmental and social factors, such as frailty and access to a toilet. Where appropriate, blood tests can be performed to assess renal function, glucose and calcium. In those patients who have haematuria or irritative symptoms, urine cytology is essential and referral to a urologist is appropriate. Additional indications requiring specialist referral are shown in Table 1.1.

Opportunities arise during routine consultations to assess not only those patients who complain of incontinence, but also those who do not present with any complaint, e.g. when there is obvious odour or wetness. Targeted questions, such as: 'Do you ever lose urine when you don't want to?', or 'Do you wear a pad or other protection to soak up urine?' are preferable to traditional enquiries, such as: 'How are your waterworks?'. During certain examinations, such as cervical cytology, post-natal examination, family planning or pelvic examination, the opportunity to evaluate pelvic floor strength arises. A simple explanation about the importance

Table 1.1. *Indications that may require specialist referral for incontinence treatment*

Uncertain diagnosis
Failure to respond to treatment
Haematuria
Recurrent urinary tract infection
Incomplete bladder emptying
Significant prolapse
Neurological problems
Vesico-vaginal fistula
Other gynaecological conditions
Previous surgery for incontinence/prostatic cancer surgery

of maintaining a healthy pelvic floor should not be missed. A basic education given early may reduce the incidence of incontinence occurring at a later stage. Male patients may be questioned during inquiries about prostatic symptoms or sexual function.

Primary health care teams should be managing patients with incontinence. Many studies have shown that conservative management in the community is highly efficacious. Bladder retraining programmes for detrusor instability indicate success rates of up to 85%, while pelvic floor exercises for GSI are successful in up to 65% of cases.[7] Early diagnosis and treatment of incontinence is the key to success, and involvement by general practitioners, practice nurses, district nurses, in association with community-based specialist nurse continence advisors, can avoid the delay caused by specialist referral. In the US, the nurse practitioner who specializes in continence care may have an affiliation through a urology or gynecology practice or may be identified by contacting continence organizations. Referral is indicated when the simple measures fail and such patients may need more sophisticated investigations, including bladder function tests, urodynamics, etc. By this means, an accurate diagnosis can be made and therapy targeted with precision. Opportunities arise during health promotion clinics and routine consultations to reinforce strategies which may prevent incontinence. Such strategies include exercise regimes, weight control, healthy diet (especially to avoid constipation), the use of hormone replacement therapy, in males, treatment of chronic cough and, in the elderly, correction of impaired mobility and adequate fluid intake. Medical management of the lower urinary tract symptoms caused by benign prostatic hypertrophy will reduce detrusor instability and the consequent urge incontinence in men, but α-blockers, used for treating hypertension, may relax the bladder neck and exacerbate incontinence, particularly in women.[8]

The primary health care teams should be managing patients with incontinence. Early diagnosis and treatment of incontinence is the key to success. Referral is indicated when the simple measures fail and such patients may need more sophisticated investigations, including bladder function tests, urodynamics, etc.

An algorithm for the shared management of patients with incontinence is shown in Fig. 1.1.[9] In the US, a urologist may have an interest in both female and male voiding dysfunction, a urogynecologist will treat only female patients. In the UK, incontinence may be investigated by any interested healthcare professional, working with appropriate facilities available to him, not necessarily a urologist or gynacologist but sometimes a geriatrician or nurse practitioner.

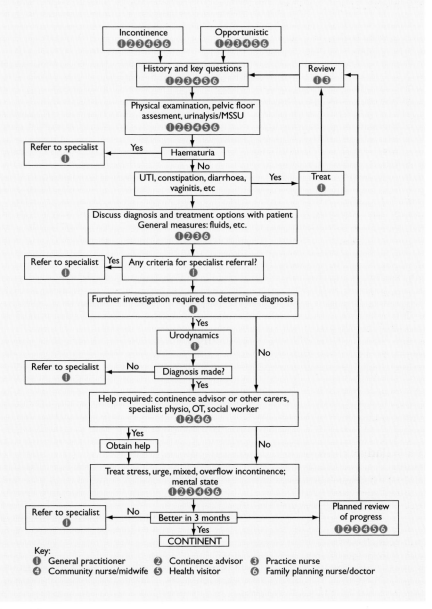

Figure 1.1.
Management of individuals with incontinence.[9] MSSU, mid stream specimen of urine.

INCREASING PUBLIC AWARENESS

In the UK and the US, there has been considerable progress in raising public awareness. Much work has been done by The Continence Foundation and The Association for Continence Advice, and as a result of this, more patients are likely to request help for the problem (see Chapter 6 for telephone helplines). Guidelines abound, but to be really useful they need to be adapted to the needs of the locality in which they are going to be used. Hilton and Stanton's algorithm[10] was the original publication indicating how to manage urinary incontinence in elderly women and much of the advice in that paper is still valid. However, a number of evidence-based national guidelines have been produced. These all offer advice on the assessment and management of incontinence due to all causes at all ages. The Agency for Health Care Policy and Research (AHCPR) urinary incontinence guidelines, published in the USA, have recently been updated[11] and are also available on the Internet in three formats (full text, short clinician's version and patient's version). The AHCPR website can be found at http://text.nlm.nih.gov:80. The Royal College of Physicians' report on the causes and management of both urinary and faecal incontinence and the provision of services is comprehensive and well referenced.[12] However, these guidelines have been written with the hospital-based clinician in mind. Primary health care guidelines, originally commissioned by the Department of Health, are now available.[13] These guidelines set out principles of good practice supported by evidence-based rationales and cover faecal as well as urinary incontinence. Adapting such guidelines to local needs can be the catalyst for communication between different professionals involved in continence care and can help clarify responsibility. Support is also provided by industry, especially pharmaceutical companies which provide educational literature for GPs.

> A number of evidence-based national guidelines have been produced including the Agency for Health Care Policy and Research (AHCPR) urinary incontinence guidelines, a report by The Royal College of Physicians' and primary health care guidelines.

THE WAY FORWARD

Traditionally, incontinence has been considered to be a nursing rather than a medical problem. There is a variable level of knowledge amongst the nursing professions, who can often manage the problem very effectively, but fail to treat the underlying cause. At the end of the day, training is the key issue and the Royal Colleges' call for incontinence education to be made compulsory in every doctor's training at undergraduate and post-graduate level. However, the immediate need is with professionals working in the community and that is where attention should be focused.

REFERENCES

1. Norton C. Increasing incontinence awareness. *J Comm Nurs* 1994; Feb: 8–12.
2. A Gallup Survey of 1423 women aged 16 to 54 (CQ 4229/A). London: Gallup, 1994.
3. O'Brien J. Evaluating primary care interventions for incontinence. *Nurs Stand* 1996, 10: 40–43.
4. Hu TW. Impact of urinary incontinence on health care costs. *J Am Geriatr Soc* 1994, 38: 292–295.
5. Brocklehurst JC. Professional and public education about incontinence. A British experience. *J Am Geriatr Soc* 1990, 38: 384–386.
6. NOP Healthcare 1997.
7. Han I, Milsom I, Fall M, Ekelund P. Long-term results of pelvic floor training in female stress urinary incontinence. *Br J Urol* 1983, 72: 421–427.
8. Agency for Health Care Policy and Research, USA. *Urinary incontinence in adults: Acute and chronic management.* AHCPR Pub no 96-0682. Rockville, MD: Dept Health and Human Services, 1996.
9. Firth J. Team practice: spend the penny wisely. *Med Mon* 1996;3 April: 63–66.
10. Hilton P, Stanton SL. Algorithmic method for assessing urinary incontinence in elderly women. *Br Med J* 1991, 282: 940–942.
11. Agency for Health Care policy and research, USA. *Urinary incontinence in adults: Clinical practice guidelines.* AHCPR Pub no 92-0038. Rockville, MD: US Dept Health and Human Services, 1992.
12. *Incontinence. Causes and management and provision of services.* London: Royal College of Physicians, 1995.
13. Button D, Roe B, Webb C *et al. Continence: Promotion and Management by the Primary Health Care team – Consensus Guidelines.* London: Whurr Publishers Ltd, 1998.

2 ANATOMY AND PHYSIOLOGY

The lower urinary tract comprises the bladder and urethra which are supported by muscles and ligaments. The bladder itself is a hollow organ composed of several layers, which include the detrusor muscle, a complex network of smooth muscle fibres and connective tissue which is responsible for bladder contractility (Fig. 2.1). On the posterior wall of the bladder, lying immediately above the bladder neck, is a small triangular area called the trigone. The two ureters enter the bladder at the uppermost angles of the trigone. At the lowermost apex of the trigone is the opening of the bladder through the bladder neck into the proximal urethra; the trigone can be identified by the fact that its epithelial lining is smooth, in contrast to the remaining bladder, which is folded into rugae.

The urethra is approximately 4–5 cm long in women and 20 cm in men. Its wall is composed of detrusor muscle interlaced with a large

> The lower urinary tract comprises the bladder and urethra. The bladder is a hollow organ composed of several layers, including the detrusor muscle which is responsible for bladder contractility.

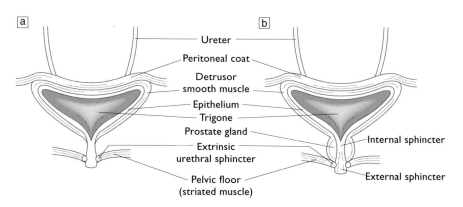

Figure 2.1.
Structure of the urinary bladder: (a) female; (b) male.

amount of elastic tissue. The prostate gland (see below) is unique to men and is situated at the bladder neck opening. The male has two functional urethral sphincters. The proximal (internal) sphincter includes the bladder neck and prostatic urethra, which extends down to the verumontanum. This area functions to prevent retrograde ejaculation in addition to continence. Transurethral resection of the prostate (TURP) has a low incidence of incontinence as the external sphincter is preserved. Radical prostatectomy for cancer may remove a portion of the intrinsic sphincter mechanism and results in a higher incidence of stress incontinence. The distal (external) sphincter extends from the verumontanum to the bulbar urethra. Women have a single urethral sphincter, which is equivalent to the male external sphincter. However, it is not as powerful as the male equivalent. The sphincter common to men and women can be divided into intrinsic and extrinsic portions (Fig. 2.2). The intrinsic part consists of epithelial, vascular, connective tissue and muscular elements. The rhabdosphincter is a circular ring of striated muscle and is thickest anteriorly, thins laterally and is virtually absent posteriorly. The muscle contains many slow-twitch fibres that are able to contract over long periods of time without fatigue. This is important in maintaining continence when at rest. The extrinsic sphincter mechanism comprises the striated muscle of the levator ani (pelvic floor) through which the urethra passes. Its fibres run laterally to the urethra, just inferior to the rhabdosphincter, and are mainly of the fast-twitch type. Consequently, they are able to contract more efficiently but over shorter time intervals, which is important during periods of exertion. The bladder neck is supported in the correct position by connective tissue and smooth muscle supports known as the pubovesical and pubourethral ligaments. These supports help to maintain the proximal two-thirds of the urethra in an intra-abdominal position. The ligaments also have an active function in the opening of the bladder neck on initiation of micturition.

> The wall of the urethra is composed of a vascular plexus and muscle interlaced with a large amount of elastic tissue. The male has two functional urethral sphincters and women have a single urethral sphincter.

The lower urinary tract is lined by transitional cell epithelium, but distally the lining of the urethra becomes stratified squamous epithelium. Beneath the epithelium is a venous plexus which contributes to urethral resistance and helps to form a watertight seal.

The prostate

An additional organ in the male called the prostate gland surrounds the urethra (prostatic urethra) (Fig. 2.3). The urethra divides the prostate into

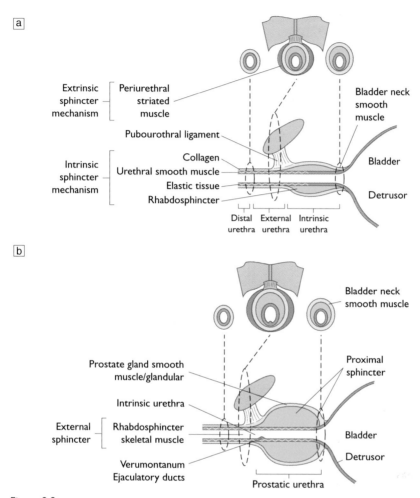

Figure 2.2.
Anatomy of the urethral sphincter: (a) female; (b) male.

an anterior fibromuscular portion and a posterior, predominantly glandular, element. The fibromuscular stroma is largely composed of smooth muscle that passes from the detrusor muscle down to the anterolateral prostate. The glandular posterolateral prostate can be subdivided into two zones – the central and peripheral zones. Although not histologically distinct

An additional organ in the male called the prostate gland surrounds the urethra (prostatic urethra).

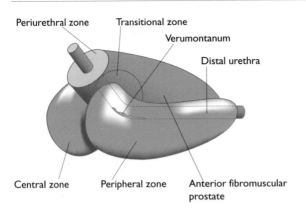

Periurethral zone   Transitional zone
                          Verumontanum
                                    Distal urethra

Central zone   Peripheral zone   Anterior fibromuscular
                                   prostate

Figure 2.3.
Three-dimensional diagram showing the anatomical relationships of the zones of the prostate.

from the peripheral zone, a smaller region of the prostate, the transition zone, lies adjacent to the urethra and extends up the bladder neck.

INNERVATION

The function of the lower urinary tract is controlled by the central nervous system via a complex system of reflex mechanisms. The cerebral cortex, brain stem and spinal cord are the main structures involved in the regulation of lower urinary tract function. The micturition cycle is thought to be initiated in the brain stem, specifically in a region known as the pontine micturition centre. This area in turn is controlled by impulses from the cerebral cortex, which has an inhibitory effect on the detrusor muscle during bladder filling.

The principle nerve supply to the bladder is via the pelvic nerves, which connect with the spinal cord through the sacral plexus, mainly S_2–S_4 (Fig. 2.4). Coursing through the pelvic nerves are both sensory nerve fibres and motor nerve fibres. The sensory fibres detect the degree of stretch in the bladder wall. Stretch signals from the posterior urethra are particularly strong and are mainly responsible for initiating the reflexes that cause bladder emptying. The motor nerve fibres transmitted in the pelvic nerves are parasympathetic. These terminate on ganglion cells located in the wall of the bladder. Short post-ganglionic nerves then innervate the detrusor muscle.

> The function of the lower urinary tract is controlled by the central nervous system via a complex system of reflex mechanisms. The principle nerve supply to the bladder is via the pelvic nerves. Sensory fibres detect the degree of stretch in the bladder wall.

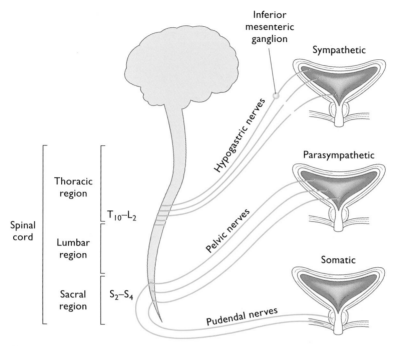

Figure 2.4.
Innervation of the lower urinary tract.

In addition to the pelvic nerves, two other types of innervation are important in bladder function. Most important are the skeletal motor fibres transmitted through the pudendal nerve to the urethral sphincter (rhabdosphincter) (Fig. 2.4). These are somatic nerve fibres that innervate and control the voluntary skeletal muscle of the sphincter. The bladder also receives sympathetic innervation through the hypogastric nerves, connecting with the T_{10}–L_2 segment of the spinal cord (Fig. 2.4). The sympathetic nervous system contributes to urine storage via relaxation of the detrusor muscle and contraction of the urethra.

NEUROPHARMACOLOGY

In parasympathetic neurons, the post-ganglionic neurotransmitter is acetylcholine, while in the post-ganglionic sympathetic neurons, the transmitter is noradrenaline (norepinephrine); the somatic nerves use acetylcholine as the neurotransmitter.

Muscarinic receptors

Contraction of the detrusor muscle is thought to be mediated primarily by stimulation of muscarinic receptors by acetylcholine and several molecularly distinct receptors have been identified. The regulation of the bladder is complex and the relative role of the various receptor subtypes in vivo remains to be clarified. The bladder contains M_2/m2 and M_3/m3 muscarinic receptors and although the M_2/m2 type predominate (80% of the total population), it is thought that the M_3/m3 type mediate contraction. Muscarinic receptors are also present on adrenergic and cholinergic nerves and are involved in the release of acetylcholine.

> Contraction of the detrusor muscle is thought to be mediated primarily by stimulation of muscarinic receptors by acetylcholine.

Adrenergic receptors

There is little sympathetic innervation of the detrusor muscle. However, noradrenaline may have a role in bladder function by inhibiting parasympathetic ganglionic transmission and possibly facilitating muscle relaxation during bladder filling through activation of β-adrenoceptors. In contrast, there is rich sympathetic innervation of the base of the bladder, prostate and urethra, which plays an important role in continence via activation of α-adrenoceptors and in the treatment of benign prostatic enlargement in inhibiting adrenergic tone.

> Sympathetic innervation of the base of the bladder, prostate and urethra plays an important role in continence via activation of α-adrenoceptors.

Non-cholinergic non-adrenergic neurohormonal influences

The exact nature of the non-cholinergic, non-adrenergic innervation of the bladder is uncertain. Neurokinin-2 receptors have been shown to exist in the human bladder and stimulation with neurokinin-A results in contraction of isolated detrusor muscle strips. Prostaglandin E and $F_{2\alpha}$ have also produced contraction of detrusor strips in vitro. It has been suggested that they are involved in maintaining tone or spontaneous activity of the detrusor; they may also act as modulators of neurotransmitter release. Vasoactive intestinal polypeptide (VIP) is a peptide associated with nerves in all layers of the bladder, beneath the epithelium, around blood vessels and in muscle layers. The inhibitory effect of VIP on both bladder and smooth muscle has been demonstrated. Although decreased levels of the peptide have been recorded in patients with detrusor instability, the role of VIP remains uncertain. Neuropeptide Y is distributed within the bladder in a similar way to VIP and may also act as an inhibitory agent.

Histamine H_1 receptors have been identified in the human bladder and activation of these results in detrusor contraction. Gamma-amino butyric acid (GABA) has been isolated from many areas of the human bladder, but the highest concentrations are found in the body of the detrusor. GABA has been shown to produce dose-dependent inhibition of contractions following nerve stimulation of isolated human detrusor muscle strips.

PHYSIOLOGY

Continence is a learnt phenomenon that depends at rest on bladder compliance, intact neurological pathways and an effective intrinsic sphincter mechanism. During exertion, the correct position of the proximal urethra, the extrinsic urethral sphincter mechanism and the state of the urethral epithelium are important factors. Appropriate voiding relies on voluntary relaxation of the urethral sphincter accompanied by removal of cortical inhibition.

> Continence is a learnt phenomenon that depends on a compliant bladder, intact neurological pathways and an effective intrinsic sphincter mechanism.

Filling phase

Urine produced by the kidneys enters the bladder via the ureters at the rate of 0.5–5.0 ml/min. The pressure within the bladder (detrusor pressure) remains approximately constant throughout the filling process and during this period the pressure in the urethra must exceed that in the bladder to maintain continence (Fig. 2.5). A combination of factors allows the bladder to maintain constant bladder pressure during filling, including the elastic and viscoelastic properties of the bladder wall and activation of neuronal mechanisms that inhibit the detrusor muscle from contracting.

Storage phase

During periods of exertion, increased intra-abdominal pressure is transmitted to the bladder, which would tend to cause expulsion of urine. However, the upper two-thirds of the urethra is normally supported in an intra-abdominal position by the pubourethral ligaments, and the sphincter mechanism (particularly the extrinsic sphincter) exerts additional force. Thus, under normal circumstances, the increased pressure is also transmitted to the bladder neck and proximal urethra, maintaining continence. This is known as positive closure pressure.

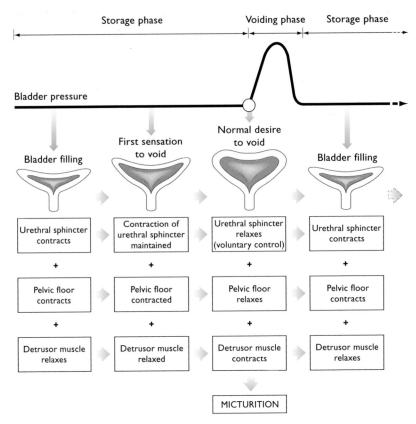

Figure 2.5.
The micturition cycle.

Voiding phase

The desire to micturate usually starts when the bladder has reached about half its physiological capacity, following which the desire to void is suppressed by the cerebral cortex until a suitable time and place for micturition has been chosen. When the micturition process is initiated, urethral pressure decreases due to voluntary relaxation of the rhabdosphincter and the pelvic floor muscles. Increased parasympathetic stimulation results in contraction of the detrusor muscle and the increase in bladder pressure leads to the voluntary initiation of micturition. Detrusor muscle contraction is maintained throughout voiding. On termination of urine flow, the bladder neck is elevated and closed through contraction of the pelvic floor; urethral pressure increases and pressure within the bladder falls. Any urine within the proximal urethra is forced ('milked') back into the bladder and bladder filling recommences.

> The micturition cycle consists of two phases: bladder filling, and storage and voiding.

3 DEVELOPMENT OF URINARY INCONTINENCE

TYPES OF INCONTINENCE

Incontinence is defined by the International Continence Society as a condition in which there is involuntary leakage of urine, which is objectively demonstrable, and is a social or hygienic problem. Urinary incontinence generally occurs if the pressure in the bladder unintentionally exceeds that within the urethra during the filling phase of the micturition cycle. There are different symptoms of urinary incontinence and these may be found in isolation or in combination. **Stress incontinence** is the involuntary loss of urine that occurs with raised intra-abdominal pressure, e.g. when coughing, laughing or exercising. **Urge incontinence** is the involuntary loss of urine which is preceded by a sudden, strong urge to void. **Mixed incontinence** is the term used to describe individuals with stress and urge incontinence. **Night-time incontinence (nocturnal enuresis)** is the involuntary loss of urine during sleep. Other forms of incontinence include **dribble incontinence**, which is the continual leakage of small volumes of urine. **Giggle incontinence** is generally confined to girls and young women (under 25 years of age) and is often self-limiting. Incontinence can occur during intercourse, either during penetration or at the time of orgasm. The distribution of different symptoms of urinary incontinence in men and women is shown in Fig. 3.1.

> Incontinence is defined as a condition in which there is involuntary leakage of urine which is objectively demonstrable and is a social or hygienic problem.

Incontinence may occur as a result of relaxation of the urethral sphincter or incompetence of the urethral closure mechanism. Other important reasons for urinary leakage include uninhibited contractions of the detrusor muscle. Causes of urinary incontinence are listed in Table 3.1.

PREVALENCE

Urinary incontinence has been estimated to affect 2–3 million individuals in the UK and around 13 million adults in the USA. Estimation of the prevalence is compromised, however, by the reluctance of people to admit

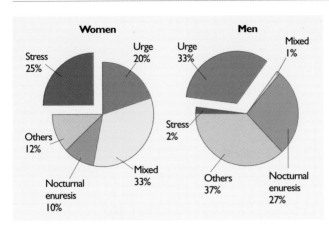

Table 3.1. *Causes of urinary incontinence*

Permanent causes	Temporary causes
● Genuine stress incontinence	● Urinary tract infection
● Detrusor instability	● Confusional states
● Voiding dysfunction	● Faecal impaction
● Neurogenic	● Oestrogen deficiency
● Congenital abnormalities	● Restricted mobility
● Urinary fistula	● Depression
● Urethral diverticulum	● Drug therapy

to urinary incontinence; many people accept it as part of their daily lives rather than seek medical attention. Variable estimates also result from differences in assessment criteria for urinary incontinence, in terms of diagnostic method and severity of urinary leakage. Nevertheless, urinary incontinence is a common problem, which affects a significant proportion of the general population (Table 3.2).

Urinary incontinence has been estimated to affect 2–3 million individuals in the UK and around 13 million adults in the USA. Overall, the incidence of urinary incontinence is higher in women than in men. Incidence also increases with age.

Overall, the incidence of urinary incontinence is higher in women than in men. Incidence also increases with age, particularly in elderly patients with psychiatric disorders.

Table 3.2. *Estimated prevalence of urinary incontinence*

	Age (years)	Prevalence (%)
Women living at home	15–44	5–7
	45–64	8–15
	≥ 65	10–20
Men living at home	15–64	3
	≥ 65	7–10
Male or female living in institutions:		
Residential homes		25
Nursing homes		40
Hospital (elderly)		50–70

GENUINE STRESS INCONTINENCE

Genuine stress incontinence (GSI) is defined as the involuntary loss of urine when the intravesical pressure exceeds the maximal urethral closure pressure in the absence of detrusor activity. GSI is the commonest cause of incontinence in women, particularly following childbirth, and can be demonstrated in 40–60% of those investigated. The symptom of stress incontinence in women is most common between the ages of 45 and 54. In general, GSI only occurs in men if they have undergone radical prostatectomy (see below) or other pelvic surgery. The incidence of incontinence associated with transurethral resection of the prostate (TURP) is approximately 1–5%, depending upon the definition of incontinence. The presence of an unstable detrusor combined with a weakened sphincter is more likely to result in post-operative incontinence.

GSI occurs as a result of a variable combination of intrinsic urethral sphincter muscle weakness and an anatomical defect in the urethral support, leading to insufficient closure pressure in the urethra during physical effort, e.g. lifting, coughing, sneezing and running. It can occur due to weakness in any component of the urethral sphincter mechanism (Table 3.3).

> GSI is defined as the involuntary loss of urine when the intravesical pressure exceeds the maximal urethral closure pressure in the absence of detrusor activity. GSI occurs as a result of intrinsic urethral sphincter muscle weakness and an anatomical defect in the urethral support.

Table 3.3. *Components of the urethral sphincter mechanism: weakness in any component can lead to genuine stress incontinence*

Supporting structure	Pubourethral ligaments
Pubovesical ligaments	
Intrinsic sphincter mechanism	Rhabdosphincter
Collagen	
Urethral vascularity (smooth muscle)	
Extrinsic sphincter mechanism	Pelvic floor musculature

The aetiology of GSI is multifactorial. Pregnancy, vaginal delivery, pelvic surgery, congenital weakness and lifestyle all contribute to its causation in women. GSI following vaginal delivery may arise due to denervation and reinnervation of the pelvic floor. Nerve damage may occur by compression or stretching. Partial damage and axon loss leads to reinnervation from remaining axons such that each axon ultimately supplies a greater number of muscle fibres. Inefficient muscle function will result, causing weakness to the pelvic floor. Pressure transmission to the proximal urethra is essential for maintenance of continence. The levator muscle contracts to support the proximal urethra and bladder base and inefficient contraction will lead to reduced pressure transmission and leakage of urine. Defects in the fascia which provide support to the urethra, as well as damage to the muscles of the pelvic floor can also contribute to GSI. Impairment of the function of the urethral sphincter may arise following trauma from surgery (e.g. hysterectomy in women; radical prostatectomy and TURP in men), instrumentation or catheterization. It is damage to the distal (external) urethral sphincter during TURP that results in incontinence, while radical prostatectomy is associated with an increased risk of damage to the distal sphincter. Male patients with stress incontinence suffer from intrinsic sphincter damage exclusively.

DETRUSOR INSTABILITY

Detrusor instability is a condition in which the detrusor is shown objectively to contract, either spontaneously or on provocation, during bladder filling whilst the subject is attempting to inhibit micturition. The characteristic symptoms are nocturia, and diurnal frequency of micturition, along with a sudden strong desire to micturate as a result of an uncontrolled detrusor contraction (urgency) and, if the contraction cannot be suppressed, urine loss (urge incontinence). Frequency occurs as a result of reduced functional bladder capacity. It is also partly a coping mechanism by the individual, which by maintaining a relatively low urinary volume in the bladder, avoids leakage of urine.

Detrusor instability is a common condition in both men and women, affecting up to 10% of the population. It is the second most common cause of urinary incontinence in women after genuine stress incontinence and is demonstrated in about 40% of women who present for urodynamic investigation. The incidence increases with age, making detrusor instability the most common cause of incontinence in the elderly.

In the majority of cases of detrusor instability, no underlying cause is found and therefore the term 'idiopathic detrusor instability' is used. Poorly learned bladder control as an infant may be the cause of detrusor instability in men or women with life-long symptoms, or maladaptive patterns of voiding may be adopted later in life. Less frequently, there is objective evidence of neurological disease, e.g. multiple sclerosis, upper motor neurone lesions due to spinal cord disruption. Detrusor instability resulting from a neurologic disorder is termed detrusor hyperreflexia (see below).

> Detrusor instability is a condition in which the detrusor is shown objectively to contract, either spontaneously or on provocation during bladder filling, whilst the subject is attempting to inhibit micturition.

There is a small increase in incidence of detrusor instability following pelvic surgery, especially after procedures for the treatment of incontinence. In men, detrusor instability may arise as a result of outflow obstruction due to benign prostatic hyperplasia (BPH) and may resolve after the obstruction has been cured.

The pathophysiology of the unstable detrusor is not fully understood. Increased sensitivity of nerve endings in the bladder to local stimuli may result in abnormal reflex responses resulting in frequency and urgency. The unstable detrusor may be caused by an upper motor neurone lesion affecting the cortical micturition centre (e.g. cerebrovascular accident). It is possible that general age-changes cause most elderly people to have some degree of bladder instability.

Many people with an unstable detrusor have no obvious neurological lesion to explain their inability to inhibit bladder contractions. This includes lifelong nocturnal enuretics (bed-wetters) and other people without overt neuropathy. It has been postulated that bed-wetting sometimes has a psychomatic cause or may be due to a congenital malformation of the bladder control centre in the brain. Another suggestion is that it arises

Symptoms of detrusor instability include: frequency, urgency and urge incontinence.

as a result of failure to learn effective subconscious bladder control. None of these explanations has been conclusively proven.

VOIDING DYSFUNCTION

Detrusor underactivity can result in the loss of effective voiding contractions. Sensation may or may not be present; if present, frequency will occur as only a small proportion of the bladder volume is used (Fig. 3.2). Sensation is often diminished and residual urine volume may become considerable (500–2000 ml), with subsequent overflow incontinence. Because of simultaneous nerve damage to the detrusor and sphincter, urethral sphincter incompetence can often coexist with detrusor underactivity. Weakness of the detrusor can result from damage to the peripheral nerves, e.g. diabetic neuropathy, or by damage to the lower spinal cord or feedback loops to the brain stem.

Detrusor underactivity can result in the loss of effective voiding contractions.

Overflow (dribble) incontinence occurs when bladder filling exceeds the functional bladder capacity. The bladder may become a large, flaccid bag, with little or no detrusor activity. Recurrent lower or upper urinary tract infections (UTIs) may occur as a result of the persistent failure to

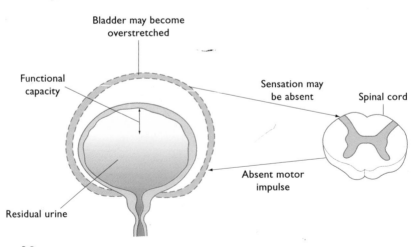

Bladder may become overstretched

Functional capacity

Sensation may be absent

Spinal cord

Absent motor impulse

Residual urine

Figure 3.2.
Underactive bladder.

completely empty the bladder, i.e. stasis of urine, which may or may not be associated with vesicoureteric reflux.

There are a number of causes of overflow incontinence (Table 3.4). Bladder injury can result from overdistension due to poor catheter management during epidural anaesthesia for obstetric delivery or surgery. The female bladder is particularly sensitive to overdistension and even one episode of acute retention of urine can result in a chronically atonic bladder. Other causes of overflow incontinence in women include prolapse and pelvic masses, e.g. fibroids.

> Overflow incontinence occurs when bladder filling exceeds the functional bladder capacity.

Table 3.4. *Causes of overflow incontinence*

Acute retention	Secondary to surgery
	Secondary to parturition
	Secondary to pain (e.g. *Herpes genitalis*)
Drugs	Diuretics
	Tricyclic antidepressants
	Anticholinergic drugs
	α-Adrenergic agonists
	Epidural analgesia
Urinary tract infection	
Urethral stricture	Surgery for genuine stress incontinence
	Urethral surgery
	Radiotherapy
Pelvic mass	Faecal impaction
	Fibroids
Detrusor hypotonia	Lower motor neurone lesions (e.g. diabetes mellitus)
Chronic myogenic failure	Connective tissue disease
	Acute retention with smooth muscle hypoxia and permanent damage
	Vascular disease

Outflow obstruction

Obstruction of the outflow of urine during voiding can lead to a variety of symptoms, including frequency, nocturia, straining to void, poor urinary stream, post-micturition dribble and urgency. In severe cases, the bladder is never completely emptied and a volume of residual urine builds up. Overflow incontinence may result (Fig. 3.3).

Outflow obstruction is most commonly associated with prostatic enlargement due to BPH, malignancy or inflammation in men.

This condition is most commonly associated with prostatic enlargement due to BPH (Fig. 3.4), malignancy or inflammation in men. Outflow obstruction in men due to prostatic enlargement, if left untreated, may result in hypertrophy of the detrusor muscle as it repeat-

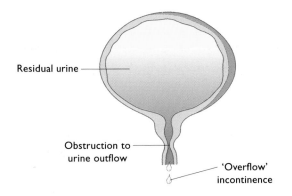

Figure 3.3.
Outflow obstruction.

Residual urine

Obstruction to urine outflow

'Overflow' incontinence

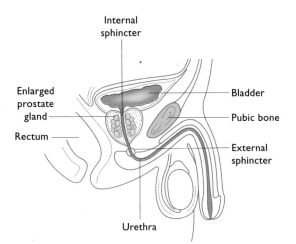

Figure 3.4.
Benign prostatic enlargement.

Internal sphincter

Enlarged prostate gland

Rectum

Bladder

Pubic bone

External sphincter

Urethra

edly tries to overcome raised outflow resistance. Secondary detrusor instability may result in trabeculation and bladder diverticulae (weakened outpouchings between hypertrophied muscle bundles).

Outflow obstruction may also occur in either sex because of urethral stenosis or stricture (possible following instrumentation or infection of the urethra). Alternatively, a neurological lesion may prevent co-ordinated relaxation of the urethra during voiding, resulting in obstruction to the outflow of urine ('detrusor-sphincter dyssynergia'). Instead of relaxing synergistically when the detrusor contracts, the urethra is in spasm and acts as an obstruction to the passage of urine. Dysfunctional voiding is the term applied to overactivity of the urethral sphincter in the absence of neuropathy.

NEUROGENIC INCONTINENCE

Sites of neurological damage

Damage to nerve pathways at any point between the cortical bladder centre and the bladder itself can impair continence (Fig. 3.5).

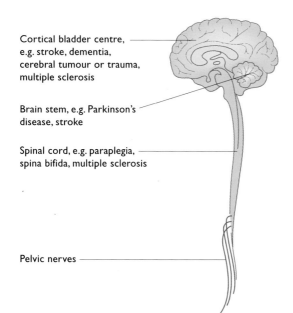

Cortical bladder centre,
e.g. stroke, dementia,
cerebral tumour or trauma,
multiple sclerosis

Brain stem, e.g. Parkinson's
disease, stroke

Spinal cord, e.g. paraplegia,
spina bifida, multiple sclerosis

Pelvic nerves

Figure 3.5.
Sites of neurological damage.

Neurolgic lesions can be divided into three functional areas: 1) infrasacral (lower motor neurone/cauda equina) or peripheral lesions occurring below the S_2-S_4 micturition reflex area located in the conus medullaris, 2) suprasacral (upper motor neurone) or spinal lesions occurring in the spinal cord between the pontine micturition centre and the micturition reflex area, and 3) suprapontine (upper motor neurone) or intracranial lesions occurring in the brain.

Peripheral nerve lesions
Subsacral lesions damaging the sacral nerve S_2-S_4 roots (cauda equina) or the peripheral nerves create a state of 'underactivity' of the bladder (areflexia) and the sphincter (denervation) mechanisms. If the extent of the lesion causes complete denervation there can be loss of the sensory (sensation of bladder filling) or motor (bladder contraction) functions of the lower urinary tract. Examples of aetiologies of infrasacral lesions can be congenital (spina bifida), inflammatory (diabetic, infectious, or nutritional neuropathy), neoplastic (sacral lipoma or metastatic breast carcinoma) lesions, or trauma (intravertebral discs, spinal stenosis, surgery or spinal anesthetic mishap, or blunt trauma). Damage to the pelvic nerve (autonomic) during extensive pelvic surgery in the female and specifically after abdomino-perineal resection for rectal carcinoma in the male can denervate the bladder. Damage to the pudendal nerve during childbirth may contribute to pelvic floor and sphincter denervation in the female.

Cauda equina lesions
Subsacral lesions damaging the sacral nerve S_2-S_4 roots create lower motor neurone bladder dysfunction. If the extent of the lesion causes denervation, then sensation of bladder filling is lost and the individual is unable to initiate micturition. Examples of subsacral lesions are protrusion of lumbosacral intervertebral discs, intradural tumours, spinal metastases, possible mishaps with epidural anaesthesia and trauma.

Spinal cord injury
The spinal shock phase that occurs following spinal cord injury is variable. During this time the bladder is areflexic and the outcome is urinary retention. As the bladder recovers, there is a return of reflex detrusor contractions, which are often poorly sustained. These, in combination with inconsistent sphincter activity, either with or without bladder neck opening, cause voiding difficulties and associated residual urine volumes.

Autonomic dysreflexia may manifest itself in patients with lesions above thoracic nerve T_5, and, in particular, it is those patients with cervical lesions who are most vulnerable during the period of spinal shock. A distended bladder, for example caused by detrusor-sphincter dyssynergia or catheter blockage, will trigger autonomic dysreflexia.

Supra-sacral spinal cord lesions
Interruptions to the pathways between the pontine micturition centre and the sacral reflex area can create a state of 'overactivity' of the bladder or 'reflex micturition' and may interrupt the bladder and sphincter coordination resulting in detrusor-sphincter dyssynergia. Congenital (spina bifida), inflammatory (multiple sclerosis, transverse myelitis), neoplastic (intrinsic and metastatic), and trauma aetiologies of spinal cord injury are possible.

Pontine micturition centre
Although pontine lesions are rare, they can result in hesitancy of micturition and urinary retention, as well as other life-threatening conditions.

Supra-pontine influences
The supra-pontine or higher centres which influence the pons are crucial for inhibiting detrusor contractions during the filling phase. Rarely, lesions in these areas, e.g. frontal lobe tumours, normal pressure hydrocephalus and cerebrovascular accidents, will result in detrusor hyperreflexia, but voiding normally remains co-ordinated as the micturition reflex (in the pons) is intact. Voluntary control of voiding – initiation or inhibition – may be lost, but the co-ordinated relaxation of the sphincter with detrusor contraction is unaffected.

> Damage to nerve pathways at any point between the cortical bladder centre and the bladder itself can impair continence.

Neurological diseases
Cerebrovascular accident
The site of the lesion will determine the type of bladder dysfunction. Detrusor hyperreflexia is a common result.

Spina bifida
The degree of damage to the lower spinal cord in spina bifida is variable and the type of bladder dysfunction depends on the amount of damage to the S_2–S_4 nerve pathways and sacral reflex area. Normal, flaccid or hyper-

reflexic detrusor muscle and a normal, flaccid, or spastic sphincter are possible options; any combination of the two is also conceivable.

Multiple sclerosis

Foci of demyelination in the brain stem or spinal cord are present in multiple sclerosis, resulting in urinary symptoms amongst others. Impaired bladder control stems mainly from the lesions in the spinal cord. Interruption between the sacral bladder centre and the pontine micturition centre results in detrusor hyperreflexia. Detrusor-sphincter dyssynergia is also possible. The most common problem is voiding difficulty in association with detrusor hyperreflexia, a combination that is difficult to treat.

Diabetes

Diseases of the peripheral nervous system can attack the local nerve supply to the bladder. This is common in diabetic peripheral neuropathy, which can affect sensory and motor pathways. With the absence of sensation, the bladder can become over-distended. Inefficient bladder emptying and overflow incontinence can result from motor damage. Detrusor instability is also possible.

Parkinson's disease

The exact nature and prevalence of bladder dysfunction in this patient group is uncertain. Detrusor hyperreflexia and striated sphincter dysfunction have been noted. As the disease progresses, the degree of voiding difficulty may increase.

CONGENITAL INCONTINENCE

Epispadias and hypospadias

Epispadias and hypospadias are congenital defects in which the urethra opens on the upper or lower surface of the penis, respectively (Fig. 3.6). Epispadias can vary from an abnormally wide meatus to a complete split of the penis; incontinence is more likely to occur with more extensive defects. With hypospadias, the urinary stream tends to pass backwards between the legs.

Epispadias can occur in girls, resulting in a short, wide urethra and stress incontinence.

Ectopic ureter

An ectopic ureter may enter the urethra directly instead of inserting into the bladder at the trigone. Continuous dribbling incontinence will result if entry to the urethra is below the urethral sphincter. Occasionally, one

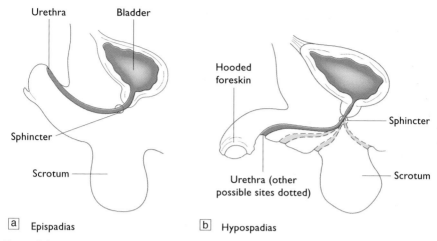

Figure 3.6.
Congenital urethral abnormality of the male. (a) epispadias, may have incontinence if proximal to sphincter. (b) hypospadias is distal to sphincter therefore no incontinence.

ureter will enter the bladder normally, whilst the other is ectopic, resulting in normal micturition as well as dribbling.

Ectopia vesicae
Ectopia vesicae is a rare congenital defect in which the bladder opens onto the anterior abdominal wall and the symphysis pubidis is separated in the midline. This condition requires early surgical correction and often results in life-long incontinence. Several attempts at surgical correction may be needed.

Urethral valve
Sometimes boys are born with dysfunctional urethral valves that prevent proper bladder emptying. This leads to retention with overflow incontinence. The child often presents with renal failure, a poor urinary stream and a UTI. This serious condition requires immediate surgical correction. The condition is now more commonly diagnosed in utero due to the use of routine ultrasound scanning during pregnancy.

A number of congenital defects can give rise to incontinence.

URINARY FISTULA

A fistula is an abnormal connection between two epithelial surfaces and in the case of urinary fistulae, it forms between the urothelium of the ureter, bladder or urethra and the epithelium of the vagina (Fig. 3.7). Sloughing of bladder or urethral tissue due to ischaemia following prolonged pressure, e.g. prolonged labour, can lead to fistula formation; infection is often a complicating factor in such cases. In the developed world, however, surgical trauma is the main cause of fistulae.

In developed countries, the most common aetiology of vesico-vaginal fistulae is gynaecological surgery, accounting for 44–74% of cases. Total abdominal hysterectomy for benign gynaecological disease is the most common surgical procedure that results in such fistulae. The most common predisposing factor is previous caesarean section. Fistulae also occur in association with pelvic malignancy or following radiotherapy. The typical presenting symptom is continuous incontinence both day and night.

Urethro-vaginal fistula is less common than the vesico-vaginal fistula, although the two may coexist. In developing countries, the major aetiological factor is childbirth, which results in ischaemic necrosis of the bladder, bladder neck and urethra. In the developed world, the main causes are anterior repair with or without vaginal hysterectomy, urethral diverticulectomy, or bladder neck suspension procedures. The site of the fistula usually dictates symptoms. Where the fistula is distal to the point of maximal urethral pressure there may be no symptoms, or there may be the symptoms of spraying of urine or post-micturition dribble as the vagina empties urine that has entered during voiding. As the site of the fistula progresses towards the bladder neck, urinary stress incontinence or recurrent UTI may become more predominant. When the fistula is proximal to the urethral sphincter mechanism, continuous incontinence is inevitable.

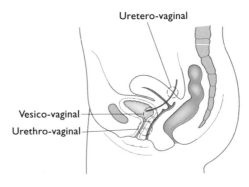

Figure 3.7.
Common sites of urinary fistulae.

Uretero-vaginal fistula is almost always the result of pelvic surgery, either direct injury with a clamp or suture, which presents early, or vascular necrosis due to excessive dissection of the ureter or the use of diathermy, in which case the lesion does not manifest itself for 10–14 days.

> Urinary fistulae can result in different symptoms of incontinence, dependent on the site of the fistula.

FAECAL IMPACTION

Severe constipation with faecal impaction can affect bladder function in various ways. Faeces in the rectum can form a physical outflow obstruction to urine by pressing on the bladder, urethra and local nerves, resulting in urinary retention with overflow of urine (Fig. 3.8). Direct pressure will also aggravate an unstable bladder. In other cases, the impaction stretches the pelvic floor inhibiting pelvic floor contractions, resulting in stress incontinence.

URINARY TRACT INFECTION (UTI)

Acute UTI can cause frequency, dysuria and transient incontinence. In the general community, the main causative organism is *Escherichia coli*, while in the hospital setting, a broad range of bacteria are implicated. Twenty

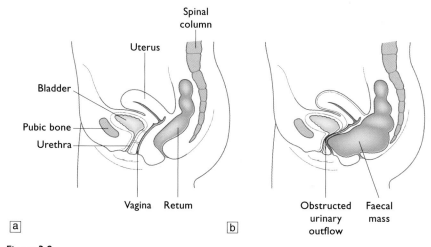

Figure 3.8.
Faecal impaction: (a) normal; (b) impacted.

percent of women will experience acute UTI at some point in their lives, while over 6% of women consult their general practitioner annually with symptoms of UTI. Recurrent UTI becomes more prevalent with increasing age. Ten percent of post-menopausal women suffer from recurrent UTI. In premenopausal women, UTI is usually associated with sexual activity, exacerbated by the use of a contraceptive diaphragm.

URETHRAL STRICTURE

Urethral stricture occurs more frequently in men than in women and results from scarred healing after an infection (urethritis) or trauma. Common sites for stricture occur either 1cm distal to the external sphincter 'bulbar urethra' or at the tip of the penis (Fig. 3.9). Symptoms include voiding difficulties, possibly with overflow incontinence and renal problems. Milder cases in females may mimic post-micturition dribble.

POST-MICTURITION DRIBBLE

Post-micturition dribble in men is the passage of small amounts of urine usually without much sensation up to several minutes after micturition is complete. This should be distinguished from terminal dribbling, which is a very slow dribbling stream at the end of micturition. The most common cause of post-micturition dribble is pooling of urine in the bulbar urethra (Fig. 3.10). The reason for an abnormally wide, lax bulb is not known. Urine can be removed by upward and forward pressure behind the scrotum. The condition can also be caused by prostatic enlargement and an

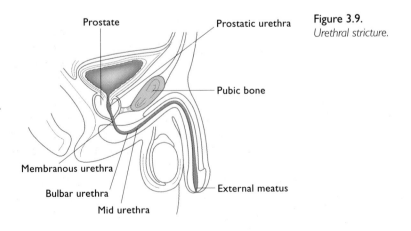

Figure 3.9.
Urethral stricture.

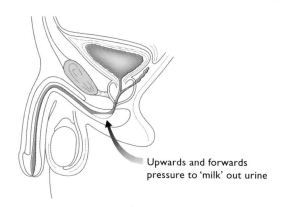

Figure 3.10.
Post-micturition dribble.

Upwards and forwards
pressure to 'milk' out urine

unstable bladder, where limited amounts or urine are forced out some-times by a powerful 'after-contraction', or with an underactive bladder.

INCONTINENCE IN THE ELDERLY

The prevalence of urinary incontinence increases with age; up to 40% of women and 22% of men over 60 years of age may be affected. With increas-ing age, there is a tendency for the bladder to be trabeculated and the detrusor muscle to become unstable, in addition to a loss of elastic tissue that supports the lower urinary tract. Chronic infection and distension makes fibrosis more common, with resulting voiding difficulties. Stress incontinence occurs more frequently in women with age as the elastic tis-sues and muscle weaken. Following the menopause, oestrogen levels decline causing alterations to the walls of the urethra that result in less efficient closure. Lack of oestrogen may also cause urethritis and trigonitis, with symp-toms of dysuria, frequency and often urgency.

> The prevalence of urinary incontinence increases with age; up to 40% of women and 22% of men over 60 years of age may be affected.

A number of medical disorders that are common in the elderly may predispose to urinary incontinence, including senile dementia, cerebrovas-cular accident, Parkinsonism, spinal-cord disease, autonomic neuropathy and endocrine abnormalities. Bladder and kidney infections are common in old age for a number of reasons. The bladder may not be emptied prop-erly, the bladder neck may be obstructed or neurological conditions may cause uncoordinated detrusor contraction with relaxation of the urethral sphincter. Most UTIs in the elderly are confined to the bladder and are low-grade and chronic. They are often associated with voiding difficulties and residual urine. BPH is the commonest form of outflow obstruction in elderly men, while underactive bladder and constipation are commonly associated with residual urine in elderly women.

Decreased mobility and limited dexterity may also contribute to incontinence. In general, anything that reduces the independence of the elderly may result in temporary urinary incontinence, e.g. acute illness, hip fracture and a change of environment, e.g. hospitalization. It is important to distinguish between transient and established incontinence in the elderly (Table 3.5), as the former are generally more amenable to therapeutic intervention.

DEVELOPMENT OF INCONTINENCE WITH AGE

Incontinence can develop during any stage of the life cycle, although certain forms of the condition are age-related as shown in Table 3.6.

Table 3.5. *Transient and established causes of urinary incontinence in the elderly*

Transient incontinence	Established incontinence
UTI (or any other infection)	Detrusor instability
Confusional states	GSI
Faecal impaction	Mixed (GSI and detrusor instability)
Restricted mobility	Voiding difficulties and overflow
Depression	
Drug therapy	

UTI = urinary tract infection; GSI = genuine stress incontinence.

Table 3.6. *Development of urinary incontinence in men and women with age*

Age	Men	Women
Birth	Epispadias/hypospadias	Ectopic ureter
	Urethral valve	Ectopia vesicae
	Ectopia vesicae	
Childhood	Bed-wetting	Bed-wetting
		Giggle incontinence
Adolescence–20 years	Detrusor instability	Intercourse incontinence
		Giggle incontinence
		UTI
20–40 years		GSI associated with childbearing
40–60 years	BPH: detrusor instability; outflow obstruction	GSI Detrusor instability
	Radical prostatectomy/TURP: GSI	
	Detrusor instability	
> 60 years	BPH: detrusor instability; outflow obstruction	Detrusor instability GSI
	Radical prostatectomy/TURP: GSI	Transient causes
	Detrusor instability	

UTI = urinary tract infection; GSI = genuine stress incontinence; BPH = benign prostatic hyperplasia; TURP = transurethral resection of the prostate.

REFERENCES

1. Feneley RCL, Shepherd AM, Powell PH *et al*. Urinary incontinence: prevalence and needs. *Br J Urol* 1979; 51: 493–496.

4 HISTORY AND EXAMINATION

The initial evaluation of a patient with urinary incontinence includes a detailed history and physical examination. The objectives of the basic evaluation are to:

- Confirm the presence of urinary incontinence
- Identify any conditions contributing to the disorder
- Decide on need for further evaluation
- Make a presumptive diagnosis if possible.

HISTORY

Urological, medical, neurological and gynaecological histories should be taken. Risk factors that are associated with urinary incontinence should also be identified and a review of medications (including non-prescription medications) made. Full details of the patient's symptoms of urinary incontinence and how they impact on lifestyle should also be obtained at this time.

> Urological, medical, neurological and gynaecological symptoms should be identified.

Urological history

The patient's normal pattern of micturition should be established. Although it is not possible to make a totally reliable diagnosis based on urinary symptoms alone, they can provide broad clues as to the likely diagnosis. The length of time the symptoms have been present can distinguish between transient and established incontinence and also whether symptoms have changed over time. A questionnaire is a useful guide as it ensures that all symptoms are enquired about; a typical one is shown in Table 4.1.

> The patient's normal pattern of micturition should be established. A questionnaire is a useful guide as it ensures that all symptoms are enquired about.

Symptoms can be grouped into mainly torage or emptying categories (Table 4.2).

Table 4.1. *Urinary symptoms questionnaire*

Name:	Wt:

Date:

Visit:

Frequency   – day (no. of times):
                – night (no. of times):
(0 = None; 1 = occasionally; 2 = often; 3 = always)

Stress incontinence:

Urgency:

Urge incontinence:

Wet at rest:

Wet on standing:

Wet at night:

Unaware wetness:

Pads/pants:

Poor stream:

Unable to stop flow:

Post-micturition dribble:

Strain to void:

Incomplete empty:

Cough:

Constipation:

Rectal soiling:

Pain on micturition:
(0 = none; 1 = urethral; 2 = perineal; 3 = suprapubic; 4 = loin)

Dyspareunia:
(0 = no; 1 = superficial; 2 = deep)

Frequency

Diurnal frequency is the number of times a person voids during waking hours; normal diurnal frequency is considered to be between 4 and 7 voids per day, but in an asymptomatic population, the range may be greater. Eight or more times is usually classed as abnormal. When establishing

Table 4.2. Urinary incontinence symptoms

Abnormal storage	• Frequency
	• Nocturia
	• Incontinence: urge, stress, coital
	• Nocturnal enuresis
Abnormal voiding	• Straining to void
	• Hesitancy
	• Incomplete emptying
	• Poor stream
	• Post-micturition dribble
Other	• Dysuria/bladder pain
	• Haematuria

frequency, a careful note must be made of fluid intake and types of fluids. Large quantities of tea and coffee can result in frequency or urgency, either because of fluid volume or because the caffeine content stimulates unstable bladder contractions. Alcohol also has an irritant effect on the bladder. Abnormal urinary frequency may occur for a number of reasons (Table 4.3).

Nocturia

Nocturia is the number of times a person is woken from sleep to pass urine. It is important to discriminate between being woken by bladder sensation and voiding because the person is already awake. Nocturia is a classic early symptom of prostatic enlargement in men. The majority of people do not need to void more than once during the night. Being woken to void twice or more is abnormal except in the very old, who appear to lose their normal diurnal variation of urinary excretion and produce urine at a consistent rate during a 24-hour period instead of more urine by day than at night. Poor diabetic control and peripheral (ankle) oedema may also lead to an increased number of voids during the night.

Incontinence

Stress incontinence is the involuntary loss of urine associated with an increase in intra-abdominal pressure, e.g. coughing, sneezing, running and lifting. There is no associated urgency and urine is usually lost in small amounts. The symptom of stress incontinence is usually caused by genuine

Table 4.3. *Possible causes of abnormal frequency*

1	Increased fluid intake and urine output: normal bladder capacity	● Osmotic diuresis, e.g. diabetes mellitus
		● Abnormal antidiuretic hormone production, e.g. diabetes insipidus
		● Polydipsia
		● Peripheral oedema
2	Reduced functional bladder capacity	● Inflamed bladder increased bladder sensation, e.g. acute bacterial cystitis
		● Detrusor instability
		● Habit or fear or urinary incontinence
		● Increased bladder sensation of normal bladder, e.g. anxiety
3	Reduced structural bladder capacity	● Fibrosis after infection, e.g. tuberculosis
		● Non-infective cystitis
		● Irradiation fibrosis
		● Post surgery, e.g. pelvic malignancy
		● Detrusor hypertrophy
4	Decreased urinary frequency	● Detrusor hypotonia, e.g. lower motor neurone lesion
		● Impaired bladder sensation, e.g. diabetic neuropathy
		● Reduced fluid intake
5	Bladder outflow obstruction	● Benign prostatic hyperplasia
		● Urethral stenosis
		● Detrusor sphincter dyssynergia

stress incontinence due to urethral sphincter incompetence, but may also occur in people with detrusor instability or with overflow incontinence.

Stress incontinence should be distinguished from urge incontinence which is leakage associated with a strong desire to void. The usual time between the first sensation of bladder filling and the need to empty the bladder is reduced. Sometimes the bladder may start to empty at the same time as the first sensation is perceived. The quantity of urine lost can be a few drops or a large volume; some individuals experience uncontrollable bladder emptying. Urge incontinence is commonly due to detrusor instability.

Coital incontinence occurs in women during sexual intercourse, either on penetration or during orgasm. The former is not associated with urgency and is more likely to occur in women with urethral sphincter incompetence. Leakage with orgasm is associated with urgency and is thought to be related to detrusor instability.

Nocturnal enuresis

Nocturnal enuresis is urinary loss during sleep and may be primary or secondary. Primary nocturnal enuresis starts in childhood and can persist into adulthood. The secondary form starts in adulthood for various reasons. It is important to differentiate the loss of urine when the patient wakens from sleep but cannot make it to the toilet from the loss of urine without wakening. True loss of urine 'while asleep' may be from oversedation from medication (tranquilizers) or from 'overflow' urinary leakage in a patient who is in urinary retention. Abnormal circadian secretion of antidiuretic hormone or detrusor instability may cause frequency at night, but the patient should wake unless a neurologic lesion has also significantly affected bladder sensation.

Straining to void

In patients who strain to void, the urinary stream is impaired and they may need to physically increase intra-abdominal pressure (apply pressure above the pubic bone) to empty the bladder.

Hesitancy

Hesitancy is a delay in initiating a urinary stream and is more common in men than in women. Hesitancy when voiding a full bladder may be an indication that the urethral sphincter is not relaxing when the detrusor contracts or that the detrusor muscle is not contracting effectively during voiding. In addition in men, it may be due to bladder outflow obstruction resulting from an enlarged prostate.

Incomplete emptying

This is the sensation of having urine left in the bladder after voiding. This can be due to fluid remaining in the bladder because of outflow obstruction (enlarged prostate) or detrusor instability causing after contractions. Women with prolapse, and large cystocele, can suffer from functional obstruction at the bladder neck resulting in increased residual urine volumes.

Poor stream
Urinary flow rate is dependent on the volume of urine passed and consequently should be assessed using a frequency/volume chart (see Chapter 5). Decreased urinary flow may be due to reduced voided volumes, bladder outflow obstruction and decreased bladder contractility.

Post-micturition dribble
This is the small, usually passive, leak of urine following voiding, usually occurring when clothes have been replaced. This symptom may be due to trapping of urine in the bulbar urethra in men, a urethral diverticulum in women, or detrusor instability. Where detrusor contractions occur after the completion of voiding, urgency will often accompany the urinary leakage. Post-micturition dribble should be distinguished from terminal dribble, which is the continuous flow of urine after the main flow and can be caused by bladder outflow obstruction due to prostatic enlargement.

Pain
Dysuria is pain or burning while passing urine and is usually due to a UTI, the urethral syndrome, or atrophic urethritis secondary to oestrogen deficiency. The urethral syndrome is the association of symptoms of frequency, urgency and dysuria in the absence of significant bacteriuria. Bladder pain more commonly occurs after micturition as the epithelium lining the bladder closes down and may be due to detrusor instability. Suprapubic pain is also associated with inflammation of the bladder, bladder stones or tumour, or some other disease process in the pelvis, such as endometriosis.

Haematuria
Blood in the urine is a serious symptom and may be indicative of a urinary tract neoplasm or stone; referral to a specialist is required. In males, it may be seen with benign prostatic hyperplasia (BHP). Microhaematuria may be secondary to a renal source, but still should be evaluated urologically.

Medical history
Any medical history that could influence bladder function or the ability to cope with it should be recorded (Table 4.4). All past major abdominal and pelvic surgery, including urinary complications, should be noted. Catheterization may have been required to treat overdistension, which can cause voiding difficulties due to detrusor hypotonia. Possible nerve damage due to a lumbar disc lesion or following spinal surgery should be con-

Table 4.4. *Medical conditions influencing bladder function*

- Major abdominal or pelvic surgery
- Chronic cough/constipation
- Cardiac/renal failure
- Endocrine disorders
- Obstetric history
- Neurological conditions
- Psychiatric disorders
- Trauma (especially spinal)

---

sidered. Operations on the large bowel, such as abdominoperineal resection of the rectum, might also have resulted in denervation. Chronic cough or constipation could be the cause of stress incontinence. Cardiac and renal failure could produce frequency and nocturia through polyuria. Endocrine disorders, such as diabetes mellitus or diabetes insipidus, might lead to polyuria and polydipsia. Chronic diabetes mellitus can produce frequency as a result of overflow incontinence secondary to a hypotonic detrusor and impaired bladder sensation.

> Any medical history that could influence bladder function or the ability to cope with it should be recorded e.g. all past major abdominal and pelvic surgery, including urinary complications, catheterization and endocrine disorders.

Obstetric history should include parity, length of labour, mode of delivery and weight of largest infant. Caesarean section or epidural block during labour and the retention of urine post partum are possible precipitators of voiding difficulties.

Neurological problems should be noted as conditions such as multiple sclerosis or multiple system atrophy can lead to detrusor hyperreflexia. Psychiatric morbidity is associated with a variety of urinary symptoms, particularly frequency, urge incontinence and nocturnal enuresis. There also appears to be an association between schizophrenia and detrusor instability.

Drug history

Many drugs have the potential to disturb lower urinary tract function, particularly those used to treat mental illness and hypertension. Major tranquillizers have an anticholinergic effect leading to voiding difficulties. Anxiolytics (benzodiazepines) and α-blockers may impair urethral

A drug history should be taken, as many drugs have the potential to disturb lower urinary tract function.

closure and exacerbate stress incontinence. Diuretics can worsen urinary frequency and urgency by increasing the rate of bladder filling (Table 4.5).

Quality of life assessment

Urinary incontinence results in impairment in many aspect of the quality of life of sufferers. The impact of incontinence on a woman's working, family and sexual life may be dramatic. Embarrassment may result in her becoming virtually housebound and unable to continue working. Coital incontinence may lead to a fear of intercourse and result in marital problems. Incontinence in men can also severely effect working and social practices. Urinary symptoms such as frequency experienced by men with BPH have been shown to limit their daily living activities and restrict places they may visit, such as the cinema and places requiring long car journeys.

It is impossible to predict on the basis of urinary symptoms and urodynamic diagnosis alone the degree of this impairment. How an individual

Table 4.5. *Examples of drugs affecting lower urinary tract function*

Drug group	Mechanism	Examples
Diuretics	Increase rate of bladder filling: exacerbate frequency and urgency	Thiazides Frusemide
β-blockers	Reduce sympathetic supply to detrusor: may enhance contractility	Atenolol Propranolol
α-blockers	Reduce sympathetic supply to urethra: decreases urethral resistance	Prazosin
Major tranquillizers	Anticholinergic effect: inhibit bladder	Chlorpromazine
Anxiolytics	Impair urethral function	Benzodiazepines
Anticholinergics	Increase urethral sphincter tone and decrease bladder contractility: urinary retention	Benzhexol Propantheline
Calcium channel blockers	Nocturia, increased frequency	Nifedipine
Anticholinesterases	Urethral sphincter muscle relaxation: involuntary micturition	Neostigmine
Opiate analgesics	Urethral sphincter spasm: difficulties in micturition; urge incontinence	Diamorphine Morphine
Alcohol	Increased urinary frequency and urgency	
Caffeine	Diuretic activity plus detrusor over activity	

tolerates their urinary symptoms varies greatly and in order to assess the effects, quality of life should be measured. Studies have demonstrated that relatively simple quality of life questionnaires can be used to measure the impact of urinary incontinence. The International Prostate Symptom Score is widely used in clinical practice for men, while the King's Health Questionnaire has been validated for women in 26 languages and has also been validated for men.

EXAMINATION

A full medical assessment should be conducted including neurological, abdominal, gynaecological and, where indicated, rectal examinations. The sign of stress incontinence in women may be identified by asking the woman to cough with a moderately full bladder, preferably while standing. It is important to perform a screening neurological examination whenever a neurological cause is a possibility, testing the tone, strength and movement of the lower limbs. It is particularly useful to test the abduction and spreading of the toes, as the innervation for the lateral abductors comes from S3. The back is examined to exclude previous spinal injury or spina bifida occulta.

> A full medical assessment should be conducted including neurological, abdominal, gynaecological and, where indicated, rectal examinations.

Abdominal examination is performed to exclude a palpable bladder or an abdomino-pelvic mass which may be pressing on the bladder. Pelvic masses such as ovarian cysts and uterine enlargement greater than that of 12 weeks' gestation can cause pressure symptoms resulting in frequency. Gynaecological examination will reveal the presence of congenital lesions such as epispadias. Examination for prolapse is essential. A profuse vaginal discharge may be the cause of apparent urinary incontinence in some women. The presence of fistula may be difficult to detect clinically and further investigation is mandatory in all suspected cases. If it is likely that a woman will need incontinence surgery, vaginal mobility and scarring should be assessed. It should be noted that women sometimes misconstrue water trapped in the vagina following a bath or swimming as urinary incontinence. This is due to the feeling of dampness when the water drains out leaving a wet patch on their underwear.

Rectal examination is particularly important in the elderly to exclude faecal impaction, which can aggravate urinary incontinence. Digital rectal examination is also important in men to assess prostatic size, shape and consistency. However, it should be remembered that chronic urinary retention due to bladder outflow obstruction can occur in the absence of any palpable enlargement of the prostate, particularly when middle lobe hyperplasia is the cause of the obstruction.

5 INVESTIGATIONS

Following the initial evaluation of the individual further investigations of lower urinary tract dysfunction may be conducted. Assessment techniques should be matched to the individual patient's needs. The basic evaluation can be carried out in the GP surgery and may include: mid-stream urine, blood tests, frequency/volume chart and pad test. Subsequent specialist investigations include urodynamic investigations, primarily uroflowmetry and cystometry, and cystourethroscopy depending on the presenting symptoms. These assess the function, rather than the structure of the lower urinary tract, and form the basis for the defining any lower urinary tract dysfunction. Additional specialized tests may also be considered.

> The basic evaluation should include: a mid-stream specimen of urine, and a frequency/volume chart. Subsequent specialist investigations include urodynamic studies, primarily uroflowmetry and cystometry, and cystourethroscopy depending on the presenting symptoms.

Mid-stream urine

A mid-stream specimen of urine is taken in order to test for conditions that are associated with or contributing to urinary incontinence, such as:

- Bacteriuria
- Pyuria
- Haematuria
- Glycosuria
- Proteinuria.

The presence of a urinary tract infection should always be checked, as such infections can invalidate the results of other investigations. A nitrate-stick test will detect the presence of bacteria in excess of 10^5/ml, indicative of an infection. Positive tests should be confirmed with urine culture, which are also necessary in determining treatment choices. If symptoms of a urinary tract infection are present in the absence of a positive culture, a

A mid-stream specimen of urine is taken in order to test for conditions that are associated with or contributing to urinary incontinence. urine sample should be sent for culture of fastidious organism, such as *Mycoplasma hominis* or *Ureaplasma urealyticum*. Dipstick methods can be used to test for the other abnormalities listed above.

Blood tests

A full blood count together with an assessment of the levels of urea, electrolytes and creatinine is performed in men to exclude the possibility of anaemia or renal impairment. A prostate-specific antigen test in men will assist in detecting BPH and prostate cancer.

Frequency/volume charts

Frequency/volume charts are used to assess voiding patterns by determining fluid intake and urine output, as well as to identify urinary incontinence and periods of urgency. Several different types of chart are available, with duration ranging from 2 to 14 days (Fig. 5.1). Information such as

Time	Day 1			Day 2			Day 3			Day 4			Day 5		
	IN	OUT	W	IN	OUT	W	IN	OUT	W	IN	OUT	W	IN	OUT	W
6am															
7am															
8am															
9am															
10am															
11am															
12															
1pm															
2pm															
3pm															
4pm															
5pm															
6pm															
7pm															
8pm															
9pm															
10pm															
11pm															
12															
1am															
2am															
3am															
4am															
5am															

Figure 5.1.
An example of a 5-day frequency/volume chart.

diurnal and nocturnal frequency, mean and maximum voided volumes, total urine output and diuresis over a 24-hour period may be extracted from the charts. These values can be used to assess the severity of symptoms. Although the ideal duration of these charts is debated, as well as the discriminative value and reproducibility of the data obtained, frequency/volume charts are widely used at the initial assessment and as follow-up to assess the efficacy of therapy. In addition, they can also indicate whether the individual is drinking too much or has an abnormal voiding pattern.

> Frequency/volume charts are used to assess voiding patterns by determining fluid intake and urine output, as well as to identify urinary incontinence and urgency.

Pad tests

Pad tests are used to verify incontinence and to quantify the degree of urine loss. The standard pad test, as recommended by the International Continence Society, involves placing a pre-weighed sanitary towel in the patient's underwear. A series of manoeuvres are then carried out by the patient over a 1-hour period, following which the pad is removed and re-weighed. Weight gain in excess of 1 g is indicative of incontinence. It is recommended that the patient drinks a 500 ml volume of fluid prior to the test. Variations to the test include different test times and instilling a standard volume of urine into the bladder prior to testing, although this turns it into an invasive test. More recently, 24- and 48-hour home pads have been suggested as these might provide more representative data.

> Pad tests are used to verify incontinence and to quantify the leakage.

Uroflowmetry

Uroflowmetry measures the rate of urinary flow during micturition and is an essential part of any urodynamic assessment. The test itself is simple, physiological and non-invasive. A variety of different methods are in use. Basically, the rate at which urine is passed is measured by a weight transducer under a cylindrical receptacle into which the patient voids (Fig. 5.2). The weight of the urine is converted electronically to give a simultaneous flow rate. In addition, the total volume of urine can be measured. As the strain gauge is measuring a change in mass, it is important to calibrate using fluid of the correct density. Other commonly used devices include a rotating disc, an electronic dip stick and the displacement of air from a container.

> Uroflowmetry measures the rate of urinary flow during micturition and is an essential part of any urodynamic assessment.

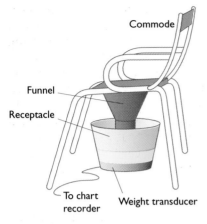

Figure 5.2.
Equipment used for uroflowmetry.

Results

Uroflowmetry is interpreted by rate and pattern. A normal pattern is characterized by a prompt start, building rapidly to a good peak and then a smooth drop (Fig. 5.3a). When the volume of urine passed is over 200 ml, a normal flow rate is at least 15 ml/s. Flow rate patterns produced by typical voiding abnormalities are shown in Figs 5.3b–d. With an underactive bladder, the pattern of voiding is unsustained as bladder emptying is by abdominal effort which can only be maintained for a few seconds at a time. In the patient with outflow obstruction, there may be a

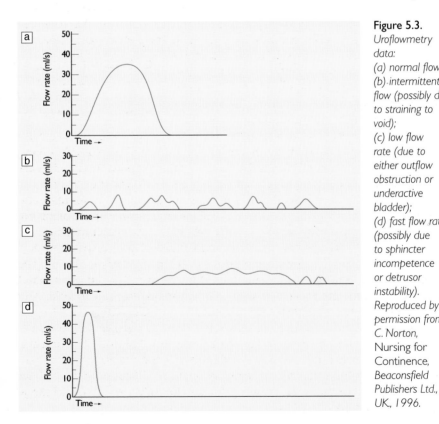

Figure 5.3.
Uroflowmetry data:
(a) normal flow;
(b) intermittent flow (possibly due to straining to void);
(c) low flow rate (due to either outflow obstruction or underactive bladder);
(d) fast flow rate (possibly due to sphincter incompetence or detrusor instability).
Reproduced by permission from C. Norton, Nursing for Continence, Beaconsfield Publishers Ltd., UK., 1996.

long period of hesitancy before the flow commences, followed by a protracted flow which may be interrupted towards the end. Although a low flow rate alone has been found to be adequate for diagnosis in 50% of men presenting with prostatic outflow obstruction, flow rate alone is not sufficient for differentiating between outflow obstruction and an underactive bladder; pressure flow studies are also required. A different flow pattern again is noted with sphincter incompetence or an overactive bladder, which is typified by a high, precipitant flow rate suggestive of low outflow resistance. It should be noted that flow rate in women is higher than in men due to lower outflow resistance caused by a shorter urethra. Also, poor flow rate prior to incontinence surgery may herald post-operative urinary retention or voiding difficulties.

Cystometry

Cystometry is the key urodynamic investigation and measures the pressure/volume relationship of the bladder. In the actual test, the patient is catheterized immediately following voiding; one catheter in the bladder is used to allow filling, while the other measures bladder (intravesical) pressure. Intra-abdominal pressure is measured through a catheter placed in the rectum or vagina. Because the bladder is an intra-abdominal organ, the detrusor is subject to changes in intra-abdominal pressure, which can lead to inaccurate diagnoses. Subtraction of intra-abdominal pressure from the intravesical pressure allows an accurate determination of the detrusor pressure.

> Cystometry is the key urodynamic investigation and measures the pressure/volume relationship of the bladder.

At the start of the investigation, the patient is asked to empty their bladder completely and the residual urine volume is measured. The bladder-filling catheter is then connected to a fluid reservoir, while the pressure catheters are connected to transducers and pressure changes recorded on a chart recorder (Fig. 5.4). The bladder is usually filled with normal saline at room temperature at the rate of 60–100 ml/min with the patient in the supine or sitting position. The first sensation of desire to void and the maximum bladder capacity are noted. The filling catheter is then removed and the patient asked to stand up and cough vigorously. Various other 'provocative' tests may be employed, such as jumping or walking on the spot, running tap water, hand washing or asking the patient to sit on the commode but not to void. Any rise in detrusor pressure or leakage is noted. The patient is then asked to pass urine into a flow meter to measure flow rate and maximum voiding pressure. During voiding the patient is requested to interrupt the flow. The urethral sphincter and pelvic floor, which are under somatic innervation, will contract immediately, but the smooth muscle of the detrusor will continue to contract for a short period of time. The resulting contraction is known as the isometric detrusor contraction.

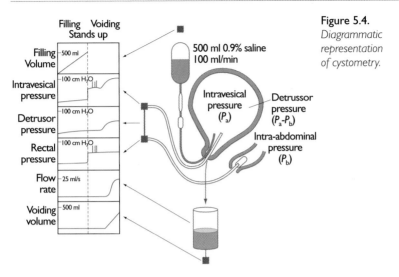

Figure 5.4.
Diagrammatic representation of cystometry.

Results

The pattern produced in a normal cystometrogram is shown in Fig. 5.5. Residual volume should be less than 50 ml; persistently large values are a sign of voiding difficulties. The normal first sensation to void occurs when the bladder contains between 150 and 250 ml; normal bladder capacity is 400–600 ml. During filling to 500 ml, the detrusor pressure does not normally rise by more than 15 cmH$_2$O. Vigorous coughing and provocative tests should not cause incontinence or bladder contractions. When the patient is instructed to void, the bladder should contract and the flow start soon afterwards. Bladder pressures inducing micturition are very variable, but are generally lower in women (30–40 cmH$_2$O) than in men (50–60 cmH$_2$O). Indeed, some women can void without a detrusor contraction. The patient should be able to stop the flow promptly by closing the sphincter and then voluntarily inhibiting detrusor contraction; the flow should be started at will.

The cystometrogram pattern in Fig. 5.6 is typical of an unstable detrusor. During the filling phase, the patient is unable to control bladder contractions and incontinence will result if bladder contractions exceed the urethral pressure. Bladder capacity is usually reduced. Detrusor pressure rises in association with the symptom of urgency are considered indicative of detrusor instability. GSI is represented in the cystometrogram as normal bladder function with incontinence during coughing (Fig. 5.7). The flow rate is normal, detrusor pressure low and the patient is often unable to

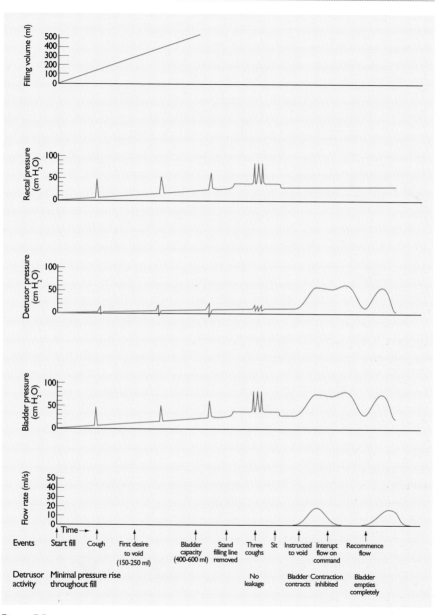

Figure 5.5.

Normal cystometrogram. Reproduced by permission from C. Norton, Nursing for Continence, *Beaconsfield Publishers Ltd., UK., 1996. (Adapted).*

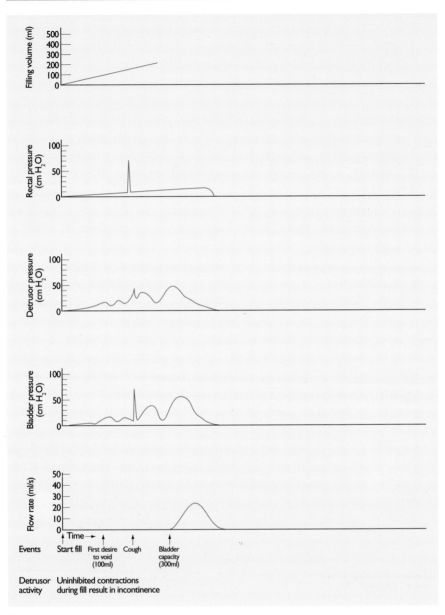

Figure 5.6.

Typical cystometrogram from a patient with an unstable detrusor. Reproduced by permission from C. Norton, Nursing for Continence, *Beaconsfield Publishers Ltd., UK, 1996. (Adapted).*

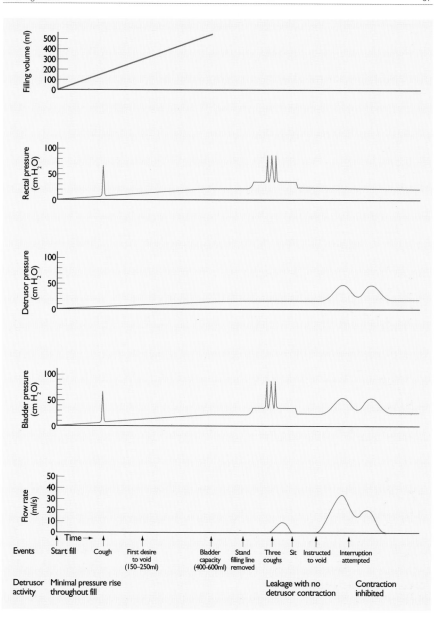

Figure 5.7.

Typical cystometrogram from a patient with genuine stress incontinence. Reproduced by permission from C. Norton, Nursing for Continence, *Beaconsfield Publishers Ltd., UK., 1996.*

interrupt the flow. Inability to interrupt the flow is very common and can occur in normal women as well as those with GSI or detrusor instability. The cystometrogram typical of a patient with an underactive bladder is shown in Fig. 5.8. The patient has no voiding contractions and any voiding that occurs is due to abdominal effort (voiding by abdominal straining) or pelvic floor relaxation. A raised detrusor pressure with reduced flow suggests a diagnosis of voiding difficulties due to outflow obstruction (Fig. 5.9).

Videocystourethrography

The lower urinary tract can be visualized during cystometry by using an X-ray screen and filling the bladder with X-ray contrast (e.g. Urografin) instead of saline. With this technique, known as videocystourethrography (VCU), the extent of bladder-base descent and leakage of contrast medium when coughing can be evaluated (Fig. 5.10). During voiding, bladder morphology can be assessed and any abnormalities noted, e.g. bladder diverticula, trabeculation and vesicouteric reflux (Fig. 5.11). Although VCU is probably the 'Gold standard' for investigation of the lower urinary tract, expense and the expertise required limit its use to a number of specialist centres. Also, it is not necessary for differentiating between GSI and detrusor instability.

The extent of bladder-base descent and leakage of contrast medium when coughing can be evaluated using videocystourethrography.

Ambulatory urodynamics

Ambulatory urodynamics measures bladder function over a longer period of time than conventional urodynamics. This technique is thought to better represent physiological conditions and be more sensitive in detecting detrusor instability. Different techniques have been described, either involving measurement of intravesical and urethral pressures or, in addition, rectal pressure over a 24-hour period (Fig. 5.12). It should be noted that this test is not yet part of the routine assessment of lower urinary tract function.

Ambulatory urodynamics measures bladder function over a longer period of time than conventional urodynamics.

Urethral pressure profilometry

Intra-urethral pressure can measured using a microtransducer catheter placed in the urethra. By slowly withdrawing the catheter, urethral pressure and intravesical pressure can be measured simultaneously though two microtip pressure transducers a set distance apart on the catheter

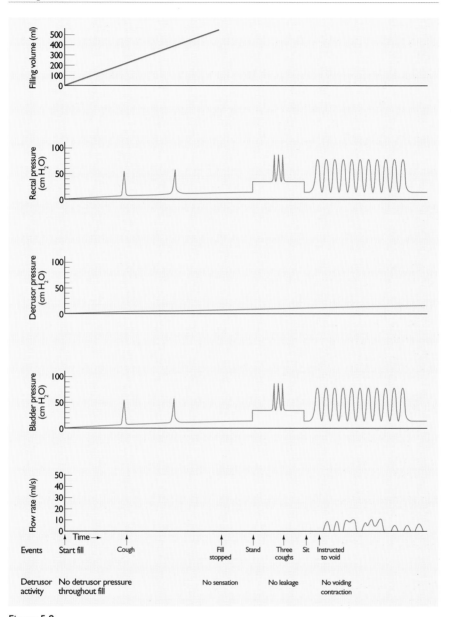

Figure 5.8.
Typical cystometrogram from a patient with an underactive bladder. Reproduced by permission from C. Norton, Nursing for Continence, Beaconsfield Publishers Ltd., UK., 1996. (Adapted).

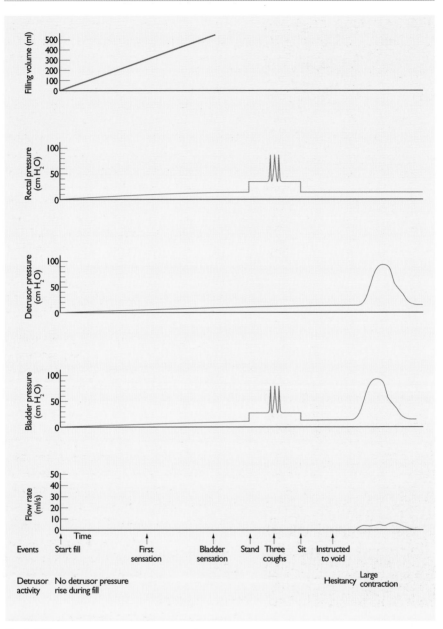

Figure 5.9.
Typical cystometrogram from a patient with outflow obstruction. Reproduced by permission from C. Norton, Nursing for Continence, *Beaconsfield Publishers Ltd., UK, 1996.*

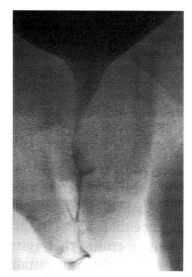

Figure 5.10.
Videocystourethrogram demonstrating bladder neck opening and urinary leakage on cough; patient subsequently diagnosed as having genuine stress incontinence.

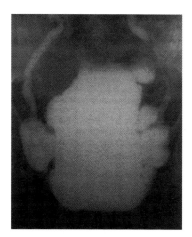

Figure 5.11.
Intravenous urogram demonstrating bladder diverticulae, trabeculation and bilateral ureteric reflux.

(Fig. 5.13). Electronic subtraction of these recordings can be made and many different parameters of the resultant trace analysed. This technique is a measure of urethral function and not detrusor function.

By asking the patient to cough repeatedly during catheter withdrawal, a cough (stress) profile can be recorded. A negative stress pressure profile is said to occur when the intravesical pressure exceeds the intra-urethral pressure during coughing. However, the size of the cough has been found to influence the stress curve, making analysis unreliable. Any fall in urethral pressure (urethral instability) can be noted by leaving the catheter in mid-urethra. This technique is not routinely used in the diagnosis of urinary incontinence, but is useful for diagnosing urethral strictures or if surgery for incontinence has failed.

> Urethral pressure profilometry is useful for diagnosing urethral strictures or if surgery for incontinence has failed.

Electromyography

Electromyography (EMG) studies the electrical potentials generated by the depolarization of the striated muscle of the urethral sphincter using needle or skin electrodes. The technique is used predominantly in patients with neuropathic disorders or in research studies.

> EMG is used predominantly in patients with neuropathic disorders or in research studies.

Ultrasonography

Ultrasound images can be obtained using the transabdominal, transvaginal, transrectal and perineal approaches. The images obtained require experience to interpret and each approach has limitations and advantages. The anatomy of the proximal urethra can be imaged and bladder volume/residual urine measured using a transabdominal approach (Fig. 5.14). As the majority of bladder cancers are exophytic and papillary in shape, they can be easily visualized on transabdominal ultrasound with a filled bladder. Other pathologies detectable using this method include bladder diverticula. The urethral sphincter can be better visualized with the transrectal or perineal ultrasound probe. Transvaginal ultra-sound images the urethral anatomy and the relationship between the urethra and the bladder neck. As the vaginal probe can easily distort the urethrovesical anatomy by pressing on the urethra, care must be taken with interpretation of results. It should be noted that incontinence cannot be diagnosed on the basis of ultrasonography alone.

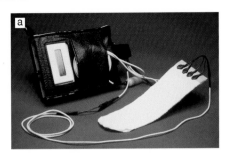

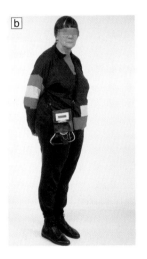

Ultrasonography can be used to detect bladder cancer and bladder diverticula.

Cystourethroscopy

Cystourethroscopy allows the visualization of the bladder and urethra with the use of a rigid or flexible cystoscope. The technique should be used if there is a history of haematuria, recurrent urinary tract infections, sensory urgency, or dysuria with normal urodynamic investigations. Bladder stones or a

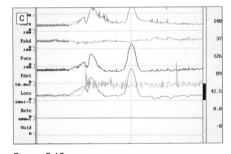

Figure 5.12.
Ambulatory urodynamic equipment: (a) alone; (b) worn by a patient; (c) the recording made.

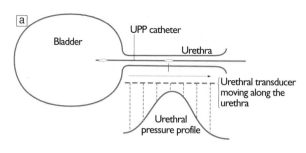

Figure 5.13.
Diagrammatic representation of urethral pressure profilometry: (a) technique; (b) a trace.

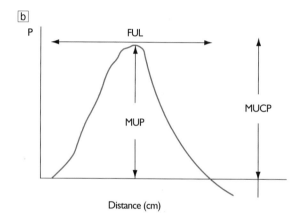

papilloma can be identified with this procedure. Other appearances to note include inflamed epithelium possibly due to chronic infection and glomerulations (petechial haemorrhages) due to interstitial cystitis. Biopsy samples can be taken, enabling the diagnosis of transitional cell carcinoma (or), interstitial cystitis or follicular cystitis. Histology can also confirm the presence of interstitial cystitis.

Cystourethroscopy should be used if there is a history of haematuria, recurrent urinary tract infections, sensory urgency, or dysuria with normal urodynamic investigations. It can identify bladder stones or a papilloma.

SUMMARY

Of the many investigations of lower urinary tract dysfunction, cystometry remains the most useful in making an accurate diagnosis. Other tests can

Of the many investigations of lower urinary tract dysfunction, cystometry remains the most useful in making an accurate diagnosis.

make useful contributions to the understanding of the underlying pathology causing lower urinary tract dysfunction. The established indications of the various tests are shown in Table 5.1.

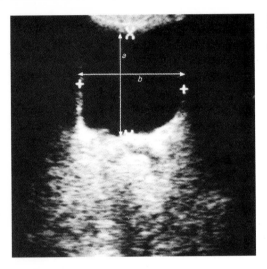

Figure 5.14.
Transverse abdominal ultrasound scan of bladder showing residual urine.

Table 5.1. *The application of investigations in diagnosing lower urinary tract dysfunction.*

	Frequency	Genuine stress incontinence	Urgency/ urge incontinence	Voiding difficulty	Fistulae
MSSU	✓		✓	✓	
Frequency/ volume chart	✓	(✓)	✓	(✓)	
Flow rate		✓		✓	
Cystometry	✓	✓	✓	✓	
VCU	✓	✓	✓	✓	✓
UPP		(✓)		✓	
EMG		(✓)		✓	
USS	✓			✓	
Cystoscopy	✓		✓	✓	✓

MSSU = mid-stream specimen of urine; VCU = videocystourethrography; UPP = urethral pressure profilometry; EMG = electromyography; USS = ultrasound scan.

6 COPING STRATEGIES

A. Billington

ADVICE

There are several helpful tips that can enable people to cope with their bladder problems, such as advice on fluid intake, diet, good bowel habit and altering voiding routines. Patients with detrusor instability may benefit most from the following advice, but it is useful for almost all those with urinary incontinence.

> Advice on fluid intake, diet, good bowel habit and altering voiding routines can enable people to cope with their bladder problems.

Fluids

It is a temptation in every incontinent person to restrict fluid intake in the hope that less fluid means less incontinent episodes. Unfortunately, this is not the case and fluid restriction may actually be counter-productive. By producing less urine the bladder is seldom stretched to full capacity, making it more sensitive to lower volumes. Restricting fluid intake also increases the tendency to constipation. However, it is also true that the more that goes in, then the more there is to come out. Fluid consumption should therefore be moderate unless there is a urinary tract infection, in which case, fluid intake should be increased. It is appropriate to advocate 1–1.5 litres of fluid per 24 hours, as this is a balance between drinking too little and drinking too much.

> It is appropriate to advocate 1–1.5 litres of fluid per 24 hours, as this is a balance between drinking too little and drinking too much.

Caffeine

Caffeine has quite a marked effect on bladder function because it is a xanthine derivative, occurring naturally in tea and coffee (particularly high concentrations occur in percolated coffee), and has a similar effect to a thiazide diuretic. It also seems to have a direct effect on the detrusor muscle causing detrusor overactivity. Caffeine appears in quite high concentrations in other drinks, such as cola drinks, Lucozade, chocolate and many slimming preparations.

Caffeine can produce lighter sleeping patterns with increased sensitivity to bladder activity. Older people are found to be more sensitive to the side-effects of caffeine, which may explain why life-long coffee drinkers may suddenly be affected. Patients are advised to avoid caffeinated drinks and food whilst undergoing a bladder retraining programme for detrusor instability. By simply avoiding caffeine, the micturition pattern will sometimes return to normal.

Caffeine can cause detrusor overactivity.

Alcohol

Alcohol can impair mobility and the perception of bladder filling. Increased urinary frequency and urgency may also result.

Diet

Patients with detrusor instability must take special care with their diet. Certain foods, such as citrus fruits and tomatoes, can make their symptoms worse, particularly in patients with interstitial cystitis. Such patients are advised to eat non-acidic fruits, such as pears and melons. Constipation should be avoided by any patient with urinary incontinence. A stool retained in the rectal vault will cause urge by pressing forward and irritating the bladder. In the patient with stress incontinence, the retained stool makes pelvic floor contraction less effective; straining during bowel movement can also undo any benefit of pelvic floor exercises. The patient should be reminded to allow time to defaecate, preferably on a daily basis. Some natural methods work as well as, if not better than, regular laxatives. The patient may find that a glass of hot water with breakfast (which should include some fruit and fibre), followed by time sitting correctly on the toilet will create a normal bowel movement. 'Natural' substances, such as sennakot or lactulose may also be beneficial.

Patients with GSI are advised not to become grossly overweight, due to the statistically significant relationship that exists between body mass index and all types of urinary incontinence. Patients who are significantly overweight and incontinent should be strongly advised to lose weight and may need referral to a dietician or a slimming club such as 'Weight Watchers'.

A number of dietary modifications are advocated including a reduction in acidic fruits.

Cranberry juice

Recurrent UTI can cause urge incontinence due to irritation. For many years cranberry juice has been recommended for reducing bacterial infection of the bladder. Studies from the 1920s and 1970s suggest that this is due to acidification of the urine. Recent research confirms that cranberry juice inhibits bacteria adherence to the bladder wall as well as *Escherichia coli* reproduction in the bowel, thereby reducing the risk of infection; it also gives some protection against yeast infection. Cranberry juice has been found to be beneficial in reducing catheter blockage for those patients with indwelling urethra or supra-pubic catheters. Patients with recurrent cystitis and bacteria should be advised to drink approximately 400 ml of cranberry juice per day, but not to drink in excess of 2 l/day as this may cause kidney stones.

> Patients with recurrent cystitis should be advised to drink approximately 400 ml of cranberry juice per day.

Toilet habit

A useful suggestion for patients presenting with bladder instability is to chart their micturition pattern for at least 1 week. This concentrates their mind on how often and why they pass urine. Once the pattern has been established, it is easier to start a bladder retraining programme, reducing the number of voids gradually by making the patient take control of their bladder again. This can be achieved by not passing urine at every opportunity, holding on whilst sitting on a hard seat if necessary, so delaying micturition by waiting for the urge to disappear. Also, patients who do not like to sit on public toilets and hover instead should be encouraged to put paper on the seat, as a proper sitting position will facilitate complete emptying. Double voiding is also recommended, because by standing up and then sitting down to try to pass urine again, the patient may empty his/her bladder completely.

Elderly patients often complain of being woken by the need to pass urine soon after falling asleep and this may simply be due to ageing. The kidneys slow down during the day but get fully perfused when the person lies down to sleep, thereby producing most urine in those first few hours of sleep. This effect can be reduced if the patient is encouraged to raise the feet to a level slightly above the heart for one hour in the afternoon and then again in the evening. Also, leg oedema is returned into the circulation when they lie down, producing more urine at night.

In many towns, incontinent patients can gain access to disabled toilets by obtaining a special key and situation guide from the local council. There are also 'urgent cards' available from The Continence Foundation to enable the incontinent person quicker access to the toilet without having the embarrassment of having to ask.

> Patients are advised to chart their micturition pattern for at least 1 week.

Clothing

Patients with incontinence should be advised about the benefits of wearing loosely fitting clothes for easy access, also the various pant and trouser adaptations and the availability of specialist clothing for patients confined to wheelchairs. Conversely, patients with stress incontinence sometimes gain some benefit from wearing tightly fitting trousers or a corset, which offers extra support to the pelvic floor, especially if there is genital prolapse. The insertion of a tampon in the vagina prior to exercise may also be helpful (see Chapter 7).

CONCLUSION

Good bladder habit should be encouraged throughout life and any urinary problem dealt with as early as possible before bad habits are formed. A continence nurse specialist is well equipped to assist the patient back to continence. Every Health District should have a Continence Advisory Service that can be contacted directly by the patient or by a Health Care Professional. To find out where your local service is contact The Continence Foundation Helpline. There are various other organizations that will be able to give advice or useful contact numbers. 'Incontact' is a patient-led organization that offers support to fellow sufferers and provide information in the form of a newsletter plus other publications. For management and equipment advice there is 'PromoCon' and for help with nocturnal enuresis, ERIC provides invaluable support and advice.

> Good bladder habit should be encouraged throughout life and any urinary problem dealt with as early as possible before bad habits are formed.

Table 6.1. *Useful contacts*

The Continence Foundation Helpline Tel: 0171 831 9831		
The Continence Foundation 307 Hatton Square 16 Baldwins Gardens London EC1N 7RJ Tel: 0207 404 6875	PromoCon Disabled Living Centre St Chad's Street Manchester M8 8QA Tel: 0161 832 3678	Simon Foundation (USA) PO Box 815 Wilmette Illinois 60091 Tel: 708 864-3913 Fax: 708 864-9758
Incontact 4 St Pancras Way London NW1 0PE Tel: 0207 717 1225	ERIC 34 Old School House Britannia Road Kingswood Bristol BS15 2DB Tel: 0117 960 3060	

7 TREATMENT OF GENUINE STRESS INCONTINENCE

INTRODUCTION

All treatment interventions for incontinence are based on the information gathered during the assessment and investigations conducted on the individual. The objective of treatment is to provide a cure by altering those factors causing incontinence. For the majority of sufferers, cure or improvement is possible, but often a series of measures may be necessary.

Treatment options including their risks, benefits and outcomes should be discussed with the individual so that informed choices can be made. As a general rule, the first choice should be the least invasive treatment with the fewest potential adverse complications.

> Treatment options for GSI can be divided into conservative measures, and surgical intervention.

Management of the condition also has to be considered and this is aimed at relieving the effects of being incontinent on the individuals and their carers. This looks at the condition in terms of quality of life and coping, and has to be considered in conjunction with treatment options.

Treatment options for GSI can be divided into conservative measures, pharmacotherapy and surgical intervention (Table 7.1).

CONSERVATIVE MEASURES

The first-line treatment for GSI involves conservative measures unless the condition is very severe. In the younger woman who has not yet completed her family, conservative therapy is used because a further pregnancy may result in a recurrence of the condition and multiple operations are often unsuccessful.

Simple measures can be instituted to improve GSI. Any precipitating or aggravating factors should be reduced as far as possible. Although increased body weight does not cause GSI, a reduction in weight may lessen the amount of leakage. Any chronic cough should be treated as this will compound the

> The first-line treatment for GSI involves conservative measures unless the condition is very severe.

Table 7.1. Treatment options for genuine stress incontinence in female patients

Conservative therapy	Pharmacotherapy	Surgery
Pelvic floor exercises	α-Adrenergic agonists	Anterior repair
Vaginal cones	(Oestrogen)	Retropubic suspensions:
Electrical stimulation	Imipramine	1. Marshall–Marchetti–Krantz
Mechanical devices		2. Burch colposuspension
		3. Laparoscopic colposuspension
		Slings
		1. Pubo-vaginal
		2. Tension-free vaginal tape
		Endoscopic bladder-neck suspension
		Periurethral injections
		Artificial urinary sphincter
		Urinary diversion

problem. Exercises that increase intra-abdominal pressure should be halted. Any constipation should also be dealt with.

In male patients with GSI, conservative measures may be taken to strengthen the external sphincter by utilizing excercises which enhance contraction of the perineal area. Stress incontinence in male patients will only be seen after surgery for benign or malignant prostatic disease which has damaged the intrinsic sphinter. Exercises which contract the anal sphincter by digital exam or electrical stimulation have been found to be useful.

Pelvic floor exercises in females

Pelvic floor exercises are the mainstay of conservative therapy for GSI. The aim of these exercises is to improve the tone of the pelvic floor muscles, in particular the levatores ani. A vaginal examination will help the patient identify the correct muscles to contract and how to achieve this. A patient-specific regimen should be established depending on the status of the muscles. Women are encouraged to perform long, slow contractions at regular intervals as well as repeated short, sharp pull-ups to enhance the strength of the fast-twitch fibres.

Pelvic floor exercises are the mainstay of conservative therapy for GSI.

A perineometer can be used to aid pelvic floor exercises (Fig. 7.1). This comprises a vaginal probe with a gauge to indicate the strength of contraction. The perineometer should not be relied upon totally as it registers when the patient bears down on it as well as when squeezing. This equipment can also be used to assess improvement in pelvic floor contractions.

Pelvic floor exercises may also benefit men who have developed urinary incontinence following radical prostatectomy or TURP.

Vaginal cones in females

Vaginal cones may be used in addition to pelvic floor exercises to improve muscle tone. They consist of a series of graded weights (20–90 g); one weight is inserted into the vagina for up to 30 minutes twice a day (Fig. 7.2). Pelvic floor contraction is essential to keep the weights in place; contracting the abdominal or gluteal muscles will not aid retention. The strength of the pelvic floor may be increased by gradually increasing the

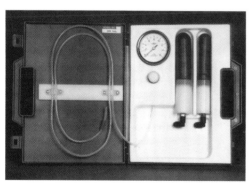

Figure 7.1.
A Bourne perineometer.

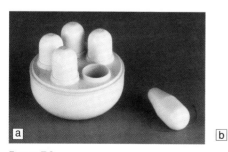
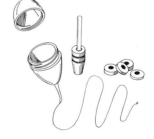

Figure 7.2.
(a) Vaginal cone; (b) parts of a vaginal cone (courtesy of The Continence Foundation).

weight of the cone. The cone is positioned just above the pelvic floor, but not too high as this may cause it to lie horizontally. The patient is encouraged to carry out normal activities, but preferably not those involving sitting. Vaginal cones are not suitable for women with a large rectocele as the cone may become trapped above the prolapse and therefore the desired therapeutic effect will be lost.

> Vaginal cones may be used in addition to pelvic floor exercises to improve muscle tone.

Electrical stimulation in females

Electrical stimulation can be applied to the pelvic floor muscles to produce contraction and to help in their re-education. Low frequency (~ 10 Hz) are thought to affect slow-twitch muscle fibres, while higher frequencies (30–50 Hz) improve fast fibre activity. A combination of the two is recommended as the pelvic floor is made up of approximately 70% slow- and 30% fast-twitch fibres.

Faradism is a technique in which a vaginal probe or plug is used to apply a direct current to the pelvic floor. This method may be uncomfortable and an alternative, commonly used technique is interferential therapy. This involves directing two high frequency voltages towards the pelvic floor from opposing directions and generating a low-frequency effect at the point of cross-over. As well as causing pelvic floor contractions, these methods assist in teaching the patient which muscle groups to contract during pelvic floor exercises.

> Electrical stimulation can be applied to the pelvic floor muscles to produce contraction and to help in their re-education.

Maximum electrical stimulation involves electrical stimulation of the pudendal nerve using vaginal or rectal plug electrodes. Stimulation of pudendal nerve afferent fibres leads to inhibition of efferent motor impulses to the bladder and results in abolition of spontaneous detrusor contractions. This procedure can be conducted at home and success rates of 30–47% have been reported.

Mechanical devices

Mechanical devices may be useful in women who have occasional incontinence associated with certain activities (e.g. sport), or who have not responded to other forms of treatment and are unsuitable for surgery. The aim of these devices is to control urinary incontinence by occluding the urethra mechanically. Mild incontinence can be controlled by the insertion of a large tampon in the lower one-third of the vagina. A commercially produced sponge tampon is available, which avoids the problem of soreness and dryness caused by continuous use of the menstrual tampon.

Another device is the foam barrier, consisting of a small triangular foam pad that has a layer of hydrophilic adhesive on one side. It is placed within the vulva and the adhesive covers the urethral meatus preventing leakage of urine. An expandable occlusive silicone device that fits inside the urethra has also been developed. Insertion is via an attached syringe and it is kept in place with a small inflatable balloon. The device is removed for voiding by pulling a short string which deflates the balloon. Early results appear promising, although the fact that the device has to be replaced after each use makes it an expensive option. It may have an application under conditions unsuited for other devices, e.g. sports. The Cunningham Clamp or occlusive foam lined clamp can be stripped around urethra to provide direct compression in males.

> Mechanical devices may be useful in women who have occasional incontinence associated with certain activities. Their aim is to occlude the urethra mechanically.

PHARMACOTHERAPY

α-Adrenergic agonists

The bladder and proximal urethra contain α-adrenergic receptors, stimulation of which results in smooth muscle contraction and an increase in the maximum urethral closure pressure. Sympathomimetic drugs with α-adrenergic agonist activity presumably cause muscle contraction in these areas, which results in increased bladder outlet resistance. The α-adrenergic agonist, phenylpropanolamine (PPA), is the first-line pharmacological therapy for women with GSI. The recommended daily dose for PPA is 25–100 mg in a sustained-release form, which is administered orally twice daily.

Analysis of clinical trials in women with GSI suggests that PPA therapy results in few cures or dryness (90–14%), but may cause subjective improvement over placebo response in 20–60% of patients. Possible side-effects include anxiety, insomnia, agitation, respiratory difficulty, headache, sweating, hypertension and cardiac arrhythmias, all of which occur more frequently in the elderly. PPA should be used with caution in patients with hypertension, hyperthyroidism, cardiac arrhythmias and angina.

Oestrogen therapy

Oestrogen can be used to improve the state of the tissues in post-menopausal women, although it is of no proven benefit in GSI. However, oestrogen does strengthen collagen fibres and so should improve the supporting ligaments of the bladder neck and the strength of pelvic floor contractions. In addition, epithelial surfaces that are better oestragenized and more vascular should facilitate urethral closure pressure by forming a water-tight seal. Oestrogen therapy is usually used in conjunction with other forms of treatment such as PPA, resulting in better results than with either drug alone.

> Oestrogen is of no proven benefit in GSI, but it can be used in conjunction with other forms of treatment such as PPA.

Imipramine

Imipramine is a tricyclic antidepressant that possesses both α-adrenergic agonist activity and anticholinergic properties and has been reported to benefit women with GSI. It is recommended as an alternative pharmacologic therapy for GSI when first-line agents have failed. Non-randomized, uncontrolled studies in small groups of women with GSI indicate continence rates of 70%. Side-effects reported include nausea, insomnia, weakness, fatigue and postural hypotension. Other drugs being developed include NS49 and β-blockers, such as propanolol.

SURGICAL INTERVENTION

The decision to perform surgery should be made only after a precise assessment has been conducted. This should include a comprehensive clinical evaluation, leading to an objective confirmation of the diagnosis of incontinence. An estimation of the impact of the proposed surgery on the patient's quality of life should also be considered. Surgery is the appropriate treatment for severe GSI or that which failed to respond to conservative therapy. It is important to make an accurate diagnosis of this condition as detrusor instability is rarely cured by surgery and, in fact, symptoms of urgency and frequency of micturition may be worsened. There are no absolute contraindications for surgery for GSI; however, relative contraindications include a neurological lesion, a chronic medical condition, or recurrent GSI following previous surgical attempts.

> Surgery is the appropriate treatment for severe GSI or that which has failed to respond to conservative therapy.

The aims of surgery are to elevate the bladder neck and proximal urethra into an intra-abdominal position where intra-abdominal pressure will act as an additional closing force. Surgery should also support the bladder neck and align it to the postero-superior aspect of the pubic symphysis which will, in some cases, increase outflow resistance. The surgical procedures for GSI that are currently in use are described below. All procedures, except where stated, relate to women.

Anterior colporrhaphy

Anterior colporrhaphy has traditionally been used to treat primary GSI in conjunction with a cystourethrocele. Although this procedure is appropriate for anterior vaginal wall prolapse, it is not really suitable for GSI. The operative technique involves a longitudinal midline incision down the anterior vaginal wall, immobilization of the bladder neck and the insertion of one or two Kelly or Pacey sutures (Fig. 7.3). The pubovesical fascia is approximated and the anterior vaginal wall closed.

Anterior colporrhaphy is relatively easy to perform and complications are rare. They include injury to the bladder, urethra and ureter, and haematoma formation; severe haemorrhage is uncommon; urinary retention may occur post-operatively. Long-term complications include recurrence of incontinence, narrowing of the vagina (which may lead to dyspareunia) and urethral stricture. A meta-analysis of 11 studies involving 957 women indicated an overall cure rate of 65% and a cure or improvement rate of 74% in the short-term. Thus, this operation has fallen into

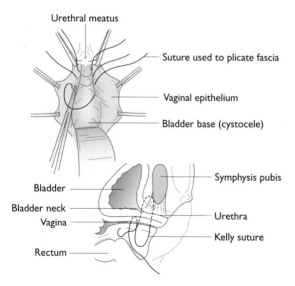

Urethral meatus

Suture used to plicate fascia

Vaginal epithelium

Bladder base (cystocele)

Symphysis pubis

Bladder

Bladder neck

Vagina

Urethra

Kelly suture

Rectum

Figure 7.3.
Technique of anterior colporrhaphy.

disrepute as treatment for genuine stress incontinence, although it remains the first line of surgery for cystocele (anterior vaginal wall prolapse).

Retropubic suspensions

Retropubic suspension procedures include several different techniques performed through a low abdominal incision (i.e. retropubic approach). All techniques have in common elevation of the lower urinary tract, particularly the urethrovesical junction within the retropubic space. The procedures differ in what structures are used to achieve the elevations. For the Marshall–Marchetti–Krantz procedure, the periurethral tissue is approximated to the symphysis pubis. While for the Burch colposuspension, the vaginal wall lateral to the urethra and bladder neck is elevated towards Cooper's ligament. A meta-analysis of 45 studies involving 3882 women undergoing these types of procedures indicated an average cure rate of 79% and a cure or improvement rate of 84%.

> Retropubic suspension procedures include several different techniques all of which include elevation of the lower urinary tract.

Marshall–Marchetti–Krantz

This procedure has been widely used for primary or recurrent GSI, although the Burch colposuspension has now superseded it. A non-absorbable suture is used to take a double bite of tissue from the bladder neck and hitch it up to the periosteum on the back of the pubic bone. The major complication is osteitis pubis (2.5–7%); bladder or urethral injury or haematoma may occur peri-operatively. In addition, this technique does not treat a cystocele.

Burch colposuspension

The Burch colposuspension is used for both primary and recurrent GSI with or without prolapse and is currently the operation of choice for this. The operation is carried out through a transverse suprapubic incision and retropubic dissection is performed to mobilize the bladder and bladder neck medially off the underlying fascia. Two to four long-term absorbable or non-absorbable sutures are inserted from the para-vaginal fascia to the ileo-pectineal ligament (Fig. 7.4).

The complications of the procedure include operative blood loss, urinary tract damage, urinary tract infection (UTI), voiding difficulties, detrusor instability and enterocele formation. UTI is common, but the incidence can be reduced by the use of a suprapubic catheter rather than a

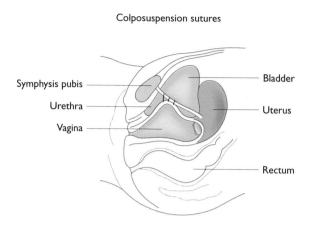

Colposuspension sutures

Figure 7.4.
*Burch colposuspension:
sagittal section showing the
final position of the bladder
neck after elevation.*

Symphysis pubis

Bladder

Urethra

Uterus

Vagina

Rectum

urethral catheter post-operatively and prophylactic antibiotics. Voiding difficulties are very common and occur in 25% of patients in the immediate post-operative period. Such difficulties can be predicted if pre-operative urodynamic assessment shows a reduced peak flow rate of less than 15 ml/s or a maximum voiding pressure of less than 15 cmH$_2$O. Late voiding difficulties following colposuspension occur in approximately 20% of those women who are identified as poor voiders pre-operatively and are associated with high pre-operative urethral resistance. Detrusor instability has been recorded in 18% of women at 3 months post-operatively; two-thirds of these women were still symptomatic after 5 years.

The Burch colposuspension is used for both primary and recurrent GSI with or without prolapse and is currently the operation of choice for this.

Laparoscopic colposuspension

Laparoscopic colposuspension is a relatively new technique which retains the principle of bladder neck and bladder base elevation, but without the need for a traditional low transverse suprapubic incision. A number of procedures have been described. The transperitoneal and retroperitoneal colposuspensions are laparoscopic versions of the Burch colposuspension. The third is a laparoscopic version of the Stamey bladder neck suspension operation and the fourth procedure involves the stapling of Prolene mesh to the paravaginal fascia and Cooper's ligament.

Laparoscopic colposuspension is a relatively new technique, with preliminary short-term high cure rates reported.

No large series has yet been reported with long-term objective follow-up; however, in a series of nearly 50 laparoscopic colposuspensions, a 90% primary cure rate was achieved. Only two randomized controlled trials have been conducted and both reported better results with laparoscopic colposuspension compared with open colposuspension.

Endoscopic bladder-neck suspension

Endoscopic bladder-neck suspension used to be advocated for primary or recurrent GSI. Nowadays, it is reserved for the old and frail in whom formal retropubic procedures may lead to higher morbidity and mortality. This procedure is easier to perform in cases where recurrent surgery has lead to scarring. Various techniques have been described, but all use two nylon sutures passed from the para-vaginal fascia to the rectus sheath or vice versa (Fig. 7.5). In the original Pereyra procedure, the sutures are passed blind, which can lead to perforation of the bladder or urethra. Additionally, misplacement of suspensory sutures has led to outflow obstruction and chronic retention. As a consequence, this procedure has become unpopular. The major modification of the Stamey procedure over that of Pereyra is the use of a cytoscope to check that the suture needle had not passed through the bladder and to ensure that it is correctly placed to elevate the bladder neck. To prevent the suspensory sutures from cutting through the pubocervical fascia, a Dacron or Silastic buffer is also used. This modification may, however, increase the incidence of infection. In the Raz procedure, sutures are placed in the endopelvic fascia and include the full thickness of the vaginal wall lateral to the bladder neck. Cytoscopy is performed to ensure adequate bladder neck elevation and to inspect for any injury to the urethra, bladder or ureters.

> Endoscopic bladder-neck suspension is reserved for the old and frail in whom formal retropubic procedures may lead to higher morbidity and mortality.

These procedures are for the most part relatively quick and easy to perform. A general anaesthetic is not mandatory since regional anaesthesia is quite adequate. Only a short hospital stay is required and a few centres have advocated the technique as a day-case procedure. The complication rate is small, but includes infection of the buffers, urinary tract damage, chronic retention and urgency. A meta-analysis of 3015 patients undergoing these types of procedures indicates that 74% of women were continent post-operatively and 84% were cured or improved. Long-term results, however, are very poor with one series reporting a 6% cure rate at 10 years.

A more recent development is the fixation of the bladder neck to the pubic bone using miniature bone anchors and a bone anchor inserter. The

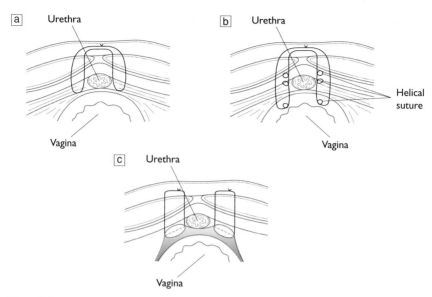

Figure 7.5.
Endoscopic bladder neck suspensions. Cross-section showing the alternative anchoring sutures: (a) modified Pereyra; (b) Raz operation; (c) Stamey procedure.

novel bone anchors are made of a shape-memory nickel titanium alloy (Nitinol) attached to Polypropylene or Gore-Tex sutures. A spring-loaded bone anchor inserter drives the anchors through the vaginal wall to a predetermined depth into the pubic bone medulla regardless of the bone's hardness, with no incision or drilling required. The device allows for the performance of a minimally invasive transvaginal bladder neck suspension with minimal morbidity. A cure rate of 82% was reported at 3 years in a small study involving 71 women; however, long-term result are not yet available. There is a risk of bone abscess or osteomyelitis with this procedure.

Slings

Sling procedures are indicated for recurrent rather than primary GSI. The advantages of such procedures are that they are useful when the urethra is scarred or the vagina is narrowed. However, slings function by causing outflow obstruction and patients need to realize that they may require clean, intermittent self-catheterization, possibly indefinitely post-operatively. Various procedures have been described involving the use of either organic material (bovine rectus sheath or strips of the patient's own rectus sheath) or inorganic material (Marlex, Mersilene, Gore-Tex or Silastic). The sling can be inserted either via an abdominal incision with retropubic dissection, or through a vaginal incision. More often, however, a combined approach is used. The sling is passed between the bladder neck and vaginal skin and is anchored either to the rectus sheath or to the ileo-pectineal ligament on either side (Fig. 7.6).

> Sling procedures are indicated for recurrent rather than primary GSI.

A recent modification of the procedure, termed 'sling on strings', uses a smaller piece of sling material with two sutures at either end, similar to those used in the endoscopic bladder neck suspension. This results in less of the expensive organic/inorganic sling material being employed. It also has the theoretical advantage of less morbidity in women who have undergone previous surgery where the dissection may be difficult. In addition, surgical trauma is less and there is a lower likelihood of perforating the bladder.

Complication rates with sling procedures are generally high and include haemorrhage, infection, injury to the bladder or urethra, erosion of the sling into the urethra, and a very significant incidence of post-operative voiding difficulties, both immediate and long term. The main problem with slings is voiding difficulties, which may be permanent, but for many urologists pubovaginal slings are the operation of first choice (not with urogynaecologists though). Data from a series of nine studies involving 434 patients with fascial slings indicated that 89% were cured and 92% were cured or improved.

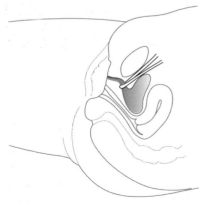

Figure 7.6.
The sling procedure.

Tension-free vaginal tape (TVT)

This technique involves using a trocar to insert Prolene tape through the anterior vaginal wall. The tape is then placed around the midurethra in a U shape and exits through two incisions made in the abdomen just above the pubic bone (Fig. 7.7). Cytoscopy is employed to ensure that the bladder has not been perforated, after which the tape is adjusted without tension under the urethra. During this adjustment the patient is asked to cough to check for continence. Consequently, the procedure is carried out under local or regional anaesthesia. A plastic sheath that covers the tape is removed and because of the strong friction that exist between the tape and the tissue canals created, no fixation of the tape is necessary. One advantage of this procedure is that the surgeon can check for continence intra-operatively without any elevation of the urethra, so avoiding post-operative urinary retention. Also the incidence of tape rejection is less than the 10% recorded with other tape materials, such as Teflon, Gore-Tex, Mersilene and Marlex.

This procedure can be carried out in under one hour on a day-care basis. High cure rates of up to 91% have been reported, but no long-term results are available as yet. Death has been reported due to inaccurate passage of the trochers through the retro-pubic space, by surgeons inexperienced in surgery for incontinence.

High short-term cure rates have been reported with TVT, but no long-term results are available as yet.

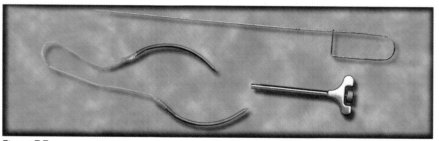

Figure 7.7.
Tension-free vaginal tape kit.

Periurethral injections

This procedure involves the injection of bulking agents such as polytetrafluorethylene (PTFE), collagen, microparticulate silicon, or autologous fat under cystoscopic guidance around the bladder neck. Patients being considered for periurethral collagen injection require a skin test for sensitivity to collagen. Injection of this material appears to be technically easier than injection of PTFE, but the longevity of PTFE versus collagen has not been

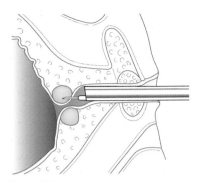

Figure 7.8.
Periurethral bulking agents.

studied. The procedure involves injection at the bladder neck in two opposing lateral planes. The collagen or silicone 'bump' can be visualized through the cystoscope and injection continues until at least 50% of the urethral lumen is occluded, after which the procedure is repeated in the opposite side (Fig. 7.8). In women, these injections can be performed under local anaesthesia.

Combined data from 15 studies of 528 women indicate that after a 2 year follow-up, 49% of patients were cured and 67% were cured or improved. Complications in women include urgency, UTI and urinary retention. Success rates in men are lower than those in women. Success is more common in men who have stress incontinence after transurethral or open prostatectomy than after radical prostatectomy. Analysis of nine studies involving 1005 men treated with periurethral injection indicated a cure rate of 20% at 2 years follow-up and a cure or improvement rate of 42%. Complications reported with the use of PTFE in men include infection, urinary retention, fever, temporary erectile dysfunction, periurethral inflammatory reaction, extrusion of the material into the urine or perineal area and burning sensation or perineal discomfort.

Particles of PTFE have been found in patients' lungs after periurethral injection, but the exact incidence and clinical significance of this migration are not known. Teflon is therefore used less frequently then collagen or microparticulate silicon, and heterologous fat usually fails.

Artificial urinary sphincter

Artificial urinary sphincters can be used in both men and women to overcome intractable stress incontinence. Suboptimal results are likely if detrusor instability or outflow obstruction are not excluded prior to surgery. Although this device is in regular use, the procedure is performed at a few, specialist centres. The technique of implantation is difficult and mechanical failure is common even with today's sophisticated devices. Additionally, these devices are very expensive.

> Artificial urinary sphincters can be used in both men and women to overcome intractable stress incontinence.

The American Medical Systems (AMS) 800 artificial urinary sphincter has been in use since 1982 (Fig. 7.9). This hydraulic device, composed of silicone rubber, has an inflatable cuff that is placed around the urethra, unidirectional valves that send liquid from a reservoir to and from the cuff and a deflation pump. Voiding is facilitated by squeezing then releasing the pump to draw liquid from the cuff into the balloon reservoir. This is repeated until sufficient liquid has been removed to allow voiding. Full repressurization of the cuff occurs automatically in about 3 min. The AMS 800 also incorporates a suspend or resume feature, which allows on–off control in the immediate post-operative period. This reduces the possibility of cuff erosion, which is thought to be caused by ischaemia secondary to compression of the vascular supply to the tissues beneath the cuff.

Female procedure
The operation involves the placement of the cuff is placed around the proximal urethra at the bladder neck. This connects to the deflation pump, which is sited in the left labia majus. The system is connected to the intra-peritoneal balloon reservoir. (Fig. 7.10).

Whilst peri-operative injury to the proximal urethra may occur, the most severe complication is erosion of the cuff through the urethra or bladder. Erosion of the pump through the skin of the labia has also been

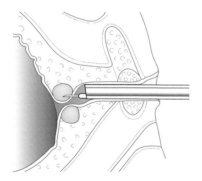

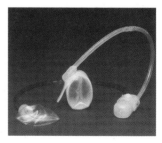

Figure 7.9. (above)
The AMS 800 artificial urinary sphincter.

Figure 7.10. (left)
The AMS 800 implanted in a female.

reported. It is likely that many of the cases of cuff erosion are due to chronic infection of the device. Erosion necessitates removal of the cuff to allow healing of the tissue defect. Re-implantation may be attempted at an interval of no less than 3 months. Success rates in highly selected groups of patients in the order of 68–100% have been reported with this technique.

Male procedure
In men, the cuff can be placed either around the urethra at the bladder neck or around the bulbar urethra (Fig. 7.11). The pump is located in the subcutaneous tunnel on one or other side of the scrotum, while the reservoir is placed in the perivesical space extraperitoneally.

As in women, the most troublesome complication is cuff erosion and device infection. One of the more common, but less significant complications of sphincter surgery is the formation of a subcutaneous haematoma. Scrotal haematomas cause most concern as they may displace the pump into an unfavourable position as well as become secondarily infected. Incomplete voiding after implantation is also possible. Analysis of 10 studies involving 346 men indicated a cure rate of 66% and a cure or improvement rate of 85%.

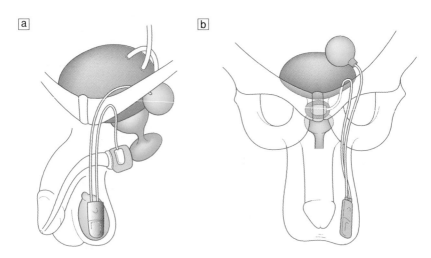

Figure 7.11.
The implanted AMS800 in a male: (a) bulbar urethra placement; (b) bladder neck placement.

Urinary diversion

Urinary diversion may be considered in women for whom all else has failed or in those with neuropathic disease. Until recently, an ileal conduit was commonly employed, but continent diversions are now undergoing evaluation. Numerous operative techniques have been developed for continent diversion of urine (Fig. 7.12). A reservoir is created from the bowel and this is emptied at intervals by clean self-catheterization through a continent abdominal valve. The frequency of catheterization obviously depends on the capacity of the reservoir (up to 1l).

> Urinary diversion may be considered in women for whom all else has failed or in those with neuropathic disease.

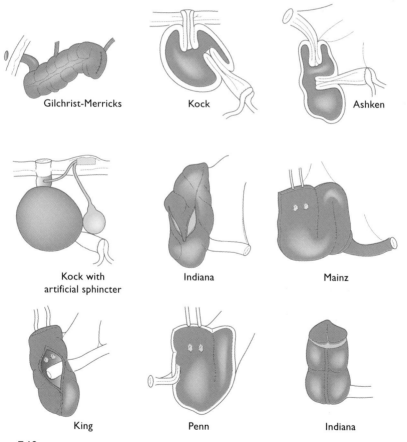

Figure 7.12.
Options for a continent urinary diversion.

8 TREATMENT OF DETRUSOR INSTABILITY

The treatment of patients with mild or intermittent symptoms associated with detrusor instability may only involve simple measures, such as reduced fluid intake, avoidance of tea, coffee and alcohol, or a change in voiding habits. More severe symptoms should be treated with methods aimed at either improving central control, such as behavioural intervention, or altering detrusor innervation, such as pharmacotherapy or, as a last resort, surgery.

PHARMACOTHERAPY

Pharmacotherapy is the mainstay of treatment for detrusor instability and a variety of agents are available.

Anticholinergic (antimuscarinic) agents

Contraction of the detrusor muscle is thought to be mediated primarily by stimulation of muscarinic receptors by acetylcholine. Consequently, a number of antimuscarinic drugs are used in the treatment of detrusor instability, e.g. oxybutinin, tolterodine, propiverine, trospium and propantheline.

Oxybutinin (Ditropan Cystrin, Dridase, Pollakisu) has both anticholinergic and direct smooth muscle relaxant properties and is currently the most commonly used drug treatment for detrusor instability. Data indicate that it effectively lowers intravesical pressure, increases bladder capacity and reduces the frequency of bladder contraction. In addition, oxybutinin has been shown to produce subjective improvements in urinary symptoms. Side-effects of this therapy are typical of anticholinergic drugs and include dry mouth (xerostomia), bad taste, dry skin, blurred vision, change in mental status, nausea and constipation. Ditropan XL, (slow release Oxybutynin) is a preparation which is already available in the US, but is also intended for future use in the UK. It has an improved side effect profile while maintaining efficacy.

Tolterodine (Detrusitol) is a muscarinic receptor antagonist that is selective for the

> Pharmacotherapy is the mainstay of treatment for detrusor instability including anticholinergic agents, muscle relaxants, antidiuretics and oestrogen.

bladder rather than the salivary glands. This results in a reduced incidence of peripheral side-effects and improved patient compliance. Several clinical trials have compared tolterodine to oxybutinin. A pooled analysis of four of these involving 1120 patients demonstrated that both drugs significantly reduced incontinent episodes and increased voided volume compared with placebo and had similar efficacy. However, oxybutinin was associated with a significantly greater frequency of adverse events, dose reductions and patient withdrawals.

Trospium (Spasmex, Spasmo-Rhoival, Spasmo-Urogenin, Trospi forte) is a quaternary anticholinergic agent indicated for the treatment of detrusor instability in several European countries (not the UK). It is reported to have a similar effect to oxybutinin in terms of its effects on urodynamic parameters. Trospium is well tolerated, but has been shown to increase the volume of residual urine in some people. Dry mouth is the most common side-effect, but generally the severity is less than with oxybutinin.

Propantheline (Pro-Banthine) is another quaternary ammonium compound with anticholinergic activity. Although not approved for use in detrusor instability, it has been reported as curing urinary incontinence in up to 5% of patients and reducing symptoms of detrusor instability in up to 53%. Anticholinergic side-effects have been reported in up to 50% of cases, with up to 9% withdrawing from treatment as a result.

Oxybutinin is currently the most commonly used drug treatment for detrusor instability.

All anticholinergic drugs are contraindicated in patients with documented narrow-angle, but not wide-angle, glaucoma.

Muscle relaxants

As noted above, oxybutinin has smooth muscle relaxant properties in addition to its anticholinergic activity. Other drugs in this category include flavoxate (Bladderon, Cistalgan, Genurin, Spasuret, Uronid, Urispas, Urispadol) which is used for the symptomatic relief of dysuria and urinary frequency associated with detrusor instability. Flavoxate is a tertiary amine with papaverine-like effect on smooth muscle. It inhibits phosphodiesterase, resulting in raised levels of cyclic adenosine monophosphate, leading to muscle relaxation. The efficacy of flavoxate in treating detrusor instability is questionable. In addition, its short half-life require a frequent dosing regimen.

Propiverine (Detrunorm, Mictonorm, Mictonetten, BUP 4) has calcium channel blocking and smooth muscle relaxing properties, as well as being a weak anticholinergic drug. It is a popular treatment for detrusor instability in Germany and in Japan. Research indicates that propiverine increases bladder capacity at both the first desire to void and when there is a strong desire to void. It also increases the voided volume at each micturition and decreases the mean frequency of micturition. However, these effects are not necessarily reflected in the clinical response to the drug. Adverse reactions are primarily related to the drug's anticholinergic properties.

Imipramine (Tofranil) is a monoamine re-uptake inhibitor (tricyclic antidepressant) with anticholinergic, anti-adrenergic, and calcium channel blocking properties. It has been shown to inhibit contractions of the detrusor muscle in vitro and to increase the tone of the smooth muscle of the bladder neck and urethra. Imipramine is associated with typical anticholinergic side-effects. If treatment is stopped abruptly, withdrawal reactions may occur, e.g. nausea, vomiting, malaise and depression (even in non-depressed individuals). The main disadvantage of imipramine is its potential for cardiotoxicity and the development of cardiac arrhythmias, probably due to the fact that the drug non-selectively blocks ion channels, including potassium ion channels in the heart. Imipramine is also associated with falls in the elderly and drowsiness, which limits its daytime use.

Antidiuretics

Desmopressin (DDAVP, Desmotabs, Desmospray, Stimate, Minirin, Minurin) is an antidiuretic and a synthetic analogue of vasopressin, but lacks the vasopressor and smooth muscle side-effects of vasopressin. It acts by inhibiting re-uptake of noradrenaline and 5-hydroxytryptamine into the presynaptic membrane, thus potentiating their action. The drug can be administered orally or intranasally. Although desmopressin is well-established in the treatment of nocturia and nocturnal enuresis, no clinical studies support its use in the treatment of detrusor instability.

Oestrogens

Oestrogen replacement may be a useful adjunctive therapy in the treatment of postmenopausal women with symptoms of detrusor instability, i.e. frequency, urgency and urge incontinence. However, no studies have shown that oestrogen therapy improves incontinence due to detrusor instability.

BEHAVIOURAL THERAPY

Bladder training

Certain cases of detrusor instability are thought to result from maladaptive learned behaviour. Treatment is therefore aimed at either 'unlearning' such behaviour or relearning a more appropriate one. The aim of bladder training, or bladder drill as it is sometimes called, is to help the patient regain control of his/her bladder by teaching him/her to resist and suppress the urge to pass urine. This will help to increase bladder capacity and to reduce the number of episodes of incontinence.

Bladder training can be carried out on an out-patient basis, but hospital admission is sometimes required to ensure that the treatment is effective. The technique involves instructing the patient to void every one and half hours during the day. Voiding must not occur in between; the patient must wait or be incontinent. The voiding interval is then increased by half an hour when the initial goal is achieved. Normal volumes of fluid are given during training.

> The aim of bladder training is to help the patient regain bladder control by teaching him/her to resist and suppress the urge to pass urine. It is effective in the short-term, but it does require a high degree of self-motivation.

Bladder training is effective in the short-term, but it does require a high degree of self-motivation. It is generally combined with other management options, such as pharmacotherapy.

Biofeedback

The aim of biofeedback is to improve bladder dysfunction by teaching people to change physiological responses that mediate bladder control. An electronic or mechanical instrument is used to relay information to the patient about their physiological activity. Single measurements using surface, needle, vaginal or anal probes can be used or multiple measurements of pelvic and abdominal/detrusor muscle activity.

Biofeedback should be used in conjunction with other behavioural techniques, e.g. pelvic floor muscle exercises, bladder training. Studies on biofeedback combined with behavioural therapy report a 54–87% improvement in incontinence across various patient groups. The biofeedback protocol associated with the greatest and most consistent symptom reduction is one that reinforces pelvic muscle contraction concurrently with inhibition of abnormal detrusor contraction; a

> The aim of biofeedback is to improve bladder dysfunction by teaching people to change physiological responses that mediate bladder control.

75–82% reduction in urinary incontinence has been reported. Biofeedback is most useful in children.

MAXIMUM ELECTRICAL STIMULATION

Maximum electrical stimulation (MES) (see Chapter 7) for detrusor instability has been shown to reduce urinary frequency and increase functional bladder capacity. Short-term home treatment with MES (20mHz frequency, 20 min/day for 12 weeks) in a limited number of women (n = 20) with detrusor instability resulted in subjective improvement in 14 women and a reduction in leakage, as judged by the pad test, in 19.

AUGMENTATION CYSTOPLASTY

Augmentation cystoplasty may be considered for cases that do not respond to other forms of treatment, and in which symptoms are severe. This major operation involves bisecting the bladder in the coronal plane anterior to the uteric orifices to within 1 cm of the bladder neck. The distance is measured and a corresponding length of ileum is isolated, opened along its antimesenteric border and sutured as a patch into the defect. This bowel segment acts by reducing the effect of the unstable detrusor contractions. Cure rates of 70% in a group of 59 patients with neuropathic bladders have been reported.

A significant risk of post-operative voiding difficulties exists, possibly as a result of diminished voiding pressures due to the ileal segment. This may be overcome by teaching the patient self-catheterization. Less commonly, urine leakage from the anastomosis and small bowel obstruction may occur. Mucus production by the bowel segment occasionally causes distress to the patient, who may have to strain to pass mucus plugs. Viscidity can be reduced with the ingestion of 200 ml daily of cranberry juice. The chronic exposure of the ileal mucosa to urine has given cause for concern with regard to possible malignant change and cases of adenocarcinoma arising in the ileal segment of have been reported. Consequently, patients undergoing this procedure need long-term follow-up and this procedure should only be used as a last resort.

> Augmentation cystoplasty may be considered for cases that do not respond to other forms of treatment and in which symptoms are severe.

URINARY DIVERSION

Urinary diversion is recommended in severe intractable cases of detrusor instability and is considered as a last resort. The technique is especially useful for young disabled patients as carers can manage a 'bag' more easily than intermittent catheterization. The technique has been described in Chapter 7.

MANAGEMENT STRATEGY

An algorithm for the management of patients with detrusor instability is shown in Table 8.1.

Table 8.1. *Management of patients with detrusor instability*

General	Decrease excessive fluid intake to 1500 ml/day
	Avoid caffeine-containing drinks and alcohol
	Supply with effective protective pads and pants
First-line intervention	Bladder retraining (alone or in combination with drug therapy)
Urge/urge incontinence	Oxybutinin
	Tolterodine
	Propiverine
	Trospium
	Oxybutinin (slow release) } (not available in the UK in January 2000)
Nocturia/nocturnal enuresis	Imipramine
	Desmopressin
Second-line intervention	Maximal electrical stimulation
Refractory cases	Augmentation cystoplasty
	Urinary diversion

9 TREATMENT OF VOIDING DISORDERS

UNDERACTIVE BLADDER (HYPOTONIC DETRUSOR)

Treatment options for underactive bladder are shown in Table 9.1.

Conservative measures

Voiding techniques

In patients with an underactive bladder due to neurological disorders, it may be possible to initiate a detrusor contraction by stimulation of certain 'trigger areas'. Elements of the sacral reflex, even though they are uncoordinated, need to be intact. Suprapubic tapping of the abdominal wall firmly and repeatedly with extended finger tips until voiding commences is a common technique. The contraction that is initiated is often unsustained, so repeated tapping may be necessary to empty the bladder; repeated tapping is also required if the reflex is weak. This process can be time consuming and frustrating for the patient. Other trigger areas that may be tried include stroking the abdomen or interior of the thigh and digital anal stimulation.

Another voiding technique is to increase abdominal pressure, particularly in women, so that urethral resistance is overcome and voluntary voiding occurs. The Valsalva and Crede manoeuvres are suitable for

Table 9.1. *Treatment options for underactive bladder*

Conservative	• Voiding techniques
	• Intermittent self-catheterization
Pharmacotherapy	• Betanechol chloride
	• Carbachol
	• Neostigmine bromide
	• Distigmine bromide
	• Physostigmine bromide
Surgery	• Electrical implant

patients with damage at the sacral bladder centre level, with low sphincter resistance. The Valsalva manoeuvre, which involves inhaling deeply and exhaling forcefully with a closed glottis, increases intra-abdominal pressure and may allow bladder emptying with straining. In certain individuals, this technique may trigger a bladder contraction. The straining employed is not recommended on a long-term regular basis, however, as it can impede cardiac return and raise intracranial pressure. Eventually, straining may weaken and damage the pelvic floor musculature and the bladder neck, resulting in sphincter incompetence and prolapse in women.

The Crede manoeuvre involves applying manual pressure with the ball of the hand to the suprapubic region over the bladder. This allows bladder emptying by either triggering a detrusor contraction or raising bladder pressure. Again, sphincter damage is a possibility if no contraction occurs and the bladder neck staysclosed.

A number of voiding techniques that stimulate a detrusor contraction can be used, such as increasing abdominal pressure.

Intermittent self-catheterization

Intermittent self-catheterization has revolutionized the treatment of patients with intractable voiding difficulty. It usually requires the patient to be both reasonably dextrous and mobile, although with additional equipment, quadriplegics may be able to perform the technique. The risk of urinary tract infection in patients with a chronic residual urine is dramatically decreased with intermittent self-catheterization.

There are two important physiological criteria in selecting patients for this procedure:

- A consistent residual urine volume greater than 100 ml
- A functional sphincter mechanism.

These features are necessary in order that adequate volumes of urine are built up in between catheterizations for the technique to be worthwhile.

The patient is usually taught how to insert the catheter by a nurse or continence advisor using a clean technique and the frequency of catheterization varies according to the individual. Some people almost empty the bladder at micturition and have a slowly accumulating residual urine over a few days. Other patients in complete retention need to catheterize five to six times per day. The frequency should be sufficient to avoid incontinence and the build up of a

Intermittent self-catheterization can be used in patients with a residual urine volume greater than 100 ml.

residual urine greater than 400 ml. The catheter is carefully washed out with running water and dried after each use, and usually replaced with a new one after about 1 week. If soreness occurs with standard disposable catheters, reusable metal ones that can be sterilized in a domestic oven can be employed.

Pharmacotherapy

The use of drugs for the treatment of an underactive bladder is disappointing due to the lack of specificity of these agents for the bladder and their undesirable effects on other organs. The cholinomimetic drugs, betanechol and carbachol, and the cholinesterases, physostigmine, neostigmine and distigmine bromide, are perhaps the most extensively researched agents advocated to encourage bladder emptying. Clinically, however, these drugs are very disappointing in patients with incomplete motor neurone lesions, myogenic injury or voiding difficulty after surgery in the absence of outlet obstruction. Side-effects include nausea, vomiting, sweating, blurred vision, bradycardia and intestinal colic.

> Pharmacotherapy for underactive bladder is disappointing.

Surgery

Nerve-stimulating implants to allow successful bladder emptying have been used in patients with partial or complete cord lesions where the sacral segments of the cord have been left intact or almost so. The stimulator is implanted in the subarachnoid space and incorporates the anterior nerve roots of S_2, S_3 and S_4. A receiver is implanted over the left lower ribs and stimulation is achieved with a radiotransmitter placed over the receiver unit. Depending on the type of stimulation, bladder contraction, rectal contraction or erection may be achieved. When the stimulator is implanted, the posterior nerve roots may be cut to abolish reflex detrusor contractions, some detrusor-sphincter dyssynergia and some low compliance. The majority of patients undergoing implantation have achieved continence with remarkably reduced residual urine volumes. Urinary tract infections are less frequent and ureteric reflux is often abolished. Problems associated with the procedure include leakage of cerebrospinal fluid, mechanical failure, accidental damage to nerve roots and infection.

> Nerve-stimulating implants can be successful in patients with partial or complete cord lesions.

OUTFLOW OBSTRUCTION

Treatment options for outflow obstruction are shown in Table 9.2.

Table 9.2. Treatment options for outflow obstruction

Conservative	● Indwelling catheter
	● Intermittent self-catheterization
	● Disimpaction of faeces
Pharmacotherapy	● α_1-Blockers
	● 5α-Reductase inhibitors
Surgery	● Urethral dilatation
	● Urethrotomy
	● Prostatectomy
	● Stents

Conservative measures
Indwelling urethral catheters
An indwelling urethral catheter is indicated in cases of acute urinary retention due to outflow obstruction (Fig. 9.1). The catheter is usually kept in place until the retention has been treated or long-term if that is not possible or unsuccessful. The most commonly used urinary catheter is the Foley catheter, which usually consists of a double lumen shaft — one for urine drainage and one for inflation and deflation of the balloon — a rounded tip and two drainage eyes proximal to the balloon (Fig. 9.2). Once inserted, the catheter is connected to a sterile drainage bag. It is important to select the correctly sized catheter, which is usually determined as the smallest one that will allow drainage. For adults this will normally be a 12–16 French gauge. There should be adequate space around the catheter to allow drainage of secretions from the paraurethral glands. Blockage of these glands and subsequent infection and stricture or abscess formation may occur with too large a catheter. Overlarge catheters may also give rise to urethral pressure sores in men at either the peno-scrotal junction or the external sphincter; sloughing granuloma and stricture formation may result.

The catheter balloon keeps the catheter in position; it does not act to block the urethral meatus. The balloon is generally filled with 10 ml or 30 ml of fluid. If too large a balloon is used, bypassing or leakage of urine around the catheter may occur. A 10 ml balloon will allow all but a small volume of residual urine to escape, while a 30 ml balloon will hold back a greater volume of residual urine, which may give rise to infection.

In addition, contractions will force the residual urine out around the catheter, causing leakage. Indwelling catheters commonly give rise to urinary tract infection, particularly with long-term use.

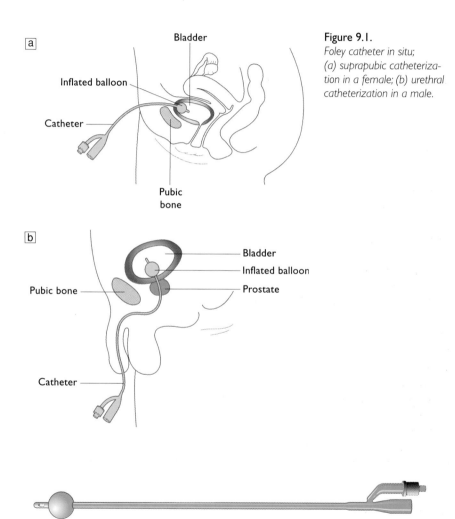

Figure 9.1.
Foley catheter in situ; (a) suprapubic catheterization in a female; (b) urethral catheterization in a male.

Figure 9.2.
The Foley catheter.

Novel catheters that lie within the prostatic urethra, but permit the external sphincter to work are currently under trial. These devices, which act more like stents than catheters, are considerably more comfortable and will hopefully reduce bacterial infection. When the catheter is no longer required, it is removed by pulling on a fine suture lying in the distal urethra. Further developments in catheter technology involve the use of biodegradable materials, which slowly dissolve over a period of weeks. This will be a major benefit to those men requiring a catheter while on a waiting list for surgery.

> An indwelling urethral catheter is indicated in cases of acute urinary retention due to outflow obstruction.

Suprapubic catheters

Suprapubic catheterization performed under local or general anaesthetic involves the insertion of a catheter through the abdominal wall just above the symphysis pubis (Fig. 9.3). This may be carried out as a temporary measure following urological or other surgical procedures, or when the patient requires long-term catheterization and is unable to carry out intermittent self-catheterization. The procedure is contraindicated if a bladder tumour is diagnosed or suspected. A variety of catheters may be used depending on cost, availability and individual preference, and includes:

- Foley
- Bonnano (Fig. 9.4)
- Stumpy Malecot
- Rutner balloon
- Pigtail
- Soft flex.

Long-term catheters should be changed at least every 8 weeks and should be 100% silicone Foleys. The initial change is normally carried out by experienced staff in the hospital setting, but subsequent changes can be undertaken by community nursing staff or trained carers or patients.

> Suprapubic catheterization may be carried out as a temporary measure following urological or other surgical procedures, or when the patient requires long-term catheterization.

Long-term complications are similar to those encountered with the urethral catheter. Additional risks include urethral leakage, especially in women, and overgranulation and bleeding at the insertion site.

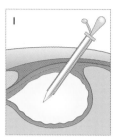 **1** Insert suprapubic introducer (trocar & sheath) into bladder, until urine can be seen rising along trocar.

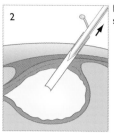 **2** Remove trocar from sheath.

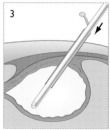 **3** Insert catheter down sheath to approximately midpoint of catheter length.

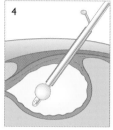 **4** Once catheter is well inside bladder, inflate balloon with 10 ml of sterile water.

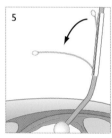 **5** Gently pull catheter to position balloon against bladder wall, then, pull off 'tear down' strip.

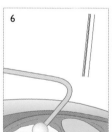 **6** Remove sheath, leaving catheter in position. (No external fixation required.)

Figure 9.3.
Procedure of suprapubic catheterization, performed under local or general anaesthetic.

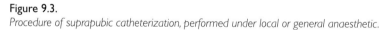

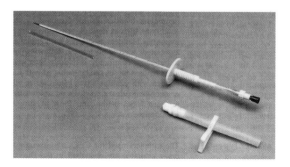

Figure 9.4.
Bonnano catheter.

Intermittent self-catheterization
See above.

Disimpaction of faeces
Outlet obstruction may occur as a result of faecal impaction and this is usually treated with daily enemas for 7–10 days. Microphosphate enemas (5–10 ml) are more comfortable for the patient, but are less effective. Once the impaction has been cleared, care should be taken to prevent reoccurrence with attention focusing on fluid intake, diet, mobility and drug regimes. Regular laxatives may be required in some patients.

Pharmacotherapy
Drugs acting on the α_1-adrenoceptors or the 5α-reductase enzyme system are useful for treatment of outflow obstruction. Established pharmacological therapy for outflow obstruction due to BPH involves these drugs either alone or in combination. α_1-Blockers act by blocking α_1-adrenoceptors in prostatic smooth muscle and the bladder neck (Fig. 9.5). As a result, they reduce outflow obstruction without adversely affecting detrusor contractility. α_1-Blockers, such as alfuzosin, terazosin, doxazosin and tamulosin, have all been shown to increase peak flow rate and improve symptoms in about 60% of patients with symptomatic BPH, i.e. incomplete emptying, frequency, intermittency, urgency, weak stream, straining and nocturia. Improvement is usually seen within 2–3 weeks. They are of little or no value in patients who are completely unable to urinate. The main side-effects of α_1-blockers are due to cardiovascular and

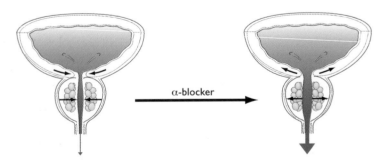

α-blocker

Figure 9.5.
Relaxation of the prostate smooth muscle and bladder neck by α_1-blockers in patients with BPH.

cerebral effects of α_1-receptor blockade. The most common side-effects are tiredness, dizziness and headache, which occur in 10–15% of patients. Postural hypotension occurs in only 2–5% of patients and this can be minimized with dose titration. It has been estimated that 13–39% of patients treated with α_1-blockers will fail therapy within 5 years.

5α-Reductase inhibitors, such as finasteride, act by inhibiting 5α-reductase, which is responsible for converting testosterone into 5α-dihydrotestosterone (DHT). DHT plays a key role in the control of prostatic growth and inhibition of 5α-reductase causes regression of the hyperplasia. Finasteride has been shown to reduce the volume of the prostate by 30% in over two-thirds of patients, with subsequent improvement in both peak urinary flow rate and symptoms. The main clinical effects of finasteride may take 3–6 months to become apparent. The efficacy of finasteride depends on prostate size, and it less effective in glands less than 40 ml. It has been show, however, to reduce the need for surgery and the incidence of acute urinary retention. The main side-effects associated with its use are reduced libido and erectile dysfunction, each occurring in 3–5% of patients; however, these effects are reversible on discontinuation of treatment.

> Drugs acting on the α_1-adrenoceptors or the 5α-reductase enzyme system relieve outflow obstruction.

Surgery

Voiding difficulty due to extrinsic urethral obstruction from an impacted fibroid uterus or a large cystocele is best treated by acute relief, i.e. catheterization, and then surgical correction of the primary abnormality. Urethral obstruction due to a calculus must be treated by its removal.

Urethral dilatation and urethrotomy

Urethral dilatation should only be undertaken when a diagnosis of outflow obstruction due to a urethral stricture (which is rare) has been made. Dilatation under local anaesthetic is difficult to achieve because of patient discomfort. Urethrotomy with longitudinal incisions of the urethral epithelium and submucosa may be more effective. Where the bladder neck has been shown to be competent, urethral dilatation does not usually cause incontinence. However, if the bladder neck is not competent, then incontinence or worsening of an existing problem may be seen.

> Urethral dilatation should only be undertaken when a diagnosis of outflow obstruction due to a urethral stricture has been made.

Table 9.3. *Indications for prostatectomy in patients with BPH*

- Acute urinary retention
- Chronic retention due to prostatic obstruction
- Recurrent urinary tract infections/haematuria
- Bladder stones secondary to BPH
- Renal insufficiency due to BPH

Prostatectomy

Prostatectomy may be necessary in patients who have complications of BPH or who have symptoms that are not controlled sufficiently by medical therapy. Specific indications for surgery are shown in Table 9.3.

Three surgical approaches are used:

- Transurethral resection of the prostate (TURP)
- Transurethral incision of the prostate (TUIP)
- Open prostatectomy.

Surgical treatment of BPH generally produces the best improvements in urinary flow rates and symptoms, but has a higher rate of complications than pharmacotherapy. The most common side-effects are retrograde ejaculation, due to bladder sphincter incompetence, and erectile dysfunction, probably due to nerve damage.

TURP

The TURP procedure is used in approximately 95% of all prostatectomies. Chips of hyperplastic tissue are excised with a diathermy loop attached to a resectoscope introduced via the urethra and removed through the resectoscope sheath (Fig. 9.6). A urethral catheter is usually retained for 36–48 hours post-operatively. TURP can improve symptoms in 70–90% of patients and increase peak flow rates to over 20 ml/s.

Urinary incontinence due to sphincter injury and urethral can occur in up to 1% of cases. Most patients also complain of dysuria and urgency of micturition for several weeks after surgery.

> Prostatectomy may be necessary in patients who have complications of BPH or who have symptoms that are not controlled sufficiently by medical therapy.

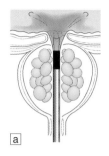
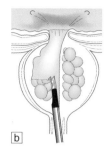
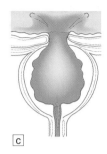

Figure 9.6.
Transurethral resection of the prostate (TURP).

Stents

Placement of a temporary or permanent stent within prostatic urethra has been used to relieve obstruction in patients with urinary retention (Fig. 9.7). They have only modest benefit, however, in men with BPH without retention. Complications associated with their use include growth of prostatic epithelium through the mesh and encrustation with calcium salts. They may also cause prolonged urethral discomfort and irritation. At present, stents remain restricted to patients in retention or those with severe obstructive symptoms who are unsuited to conventional surgery.

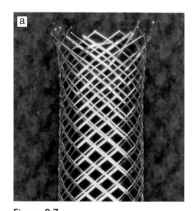
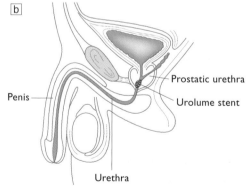

Figure 9.7.
(a) The Urolume permanent stent; (b) the Urolume stent in situ.

FISTULA

Rarely, a small vesico-vaginal fistula may heal spontaneously with prolonged bladder drainage; however, steps are needed if healing does not occur within 3–4 weeks. Controversy exists over the timing of any surgical repair. Traditionally, a 3–4 month wait has been recommended in order that complete resolution of inflammation and oedema may occur. At this time the area of devascularization is completely demarcated and there is clear delineation of fibrotic tissue. Undoubtedly, this sort of delay can be distressing to the patient and early repair, particularly if the injury is due to surgical trauma, is becoming increasingly popular.

Surgical repair can be through an abdominal, vaginal or a combined approach. An abdominal or combined approach is more appropriate under the following circumstances: large or multiple fistulae, poor vaginal access, ureteric involvement requiring other urological procedures, recurrent fistulae and the presence of poor quality tissue, e.g. following radiotherapy. Vaginal surgery is a relatively minor procedure with a short recovery time. Occasionally, however, some loss of functional vaginal length may occur as well as stress incontinence due to altered mobility of the bladder neck.

The use of a pedicle graft to provide viable tissue may be required if tissue loss is extensive. A Martius graft (subcutaneous fat pedicle from the labium majus) or a gracilis graft may be used for this purpose. Post-operatively, free bladder drainage is continued for 2 weeks, but longer for fistula secondary to irradiation. Overall success rates for primary closure are over 90%. The rates in developing countries are somewhat lower at 75%, with a further 15% following a second procedure. Results of post-irradiation fistula repair are less successful, with cure rates as low as 60%. Urinary diversion should only be performed as a last resort, and implantation of ureters into the bowel must only be undertaken if there is no recto-vaginal fistula and the anal sphincter is capable of maintaining continence of liquid faeces.

> Surgical repair of fistulae can be through an abdominal, vaginal or a combined approach.

CONGENITAL ABNORMALITIES

Treatment of congenital abnormalities is usually surgical. Some repairs are done in several stages, while less serious conditions are left until the child can cope better psychologically.

RECURRENT URINARY TRACT INFECTION

Treatment should be aimed at the underlying condition that predisposes to recurrent urinary tract infection (UTI). Incomplete bladder emptying should be adequately investigated urodynamically and treatment initiated to improve bladder contractility or reduce urethral resistance where appropriate. Constipation and faecal impaction should be dealt with, as they predispose to UTI in the elderly.

Antibiotics are indicated for the treatment of acute UTI, but their role in management of women with recurrent UTI is limited. Long-term use may also lead to bacterial resistanse, causing increased morbidity. In patients with indwelling catheters, each infection should be dealt with on an individual basis, with culture and appropriate therapy. Due to the high incidence of resistance, penicillins are no longer considered first-line treatment in simple UTI. In vitro results suggest that 20–40% of infections are resistant to trimethoprim, although clinical response is often better than this. Cephalosporins appear as effective as trimethoprim, but are associated with considerable side-effects, as is nalidixic acid.

> Treatment should be aimed at the underlying condition that predisposes to recurrent urinary tract infection.

INTERSTITIAL CYSTITIS

In addition to irritative bladder symptoms, common findings in interstitial cystitis are lower abdominal pain, perineal discomfort, dysuria and dyspareunia. The aetiology of interstitial cystitis is poorly understood and many therapeutic modalities have been tried, with varying degrees of success. A number of systemic therapies that may be beneficial are shown in Table 10.1. Local treatment involves bladder distension and installation therapy. Improvement in symptoms may be dramatic following bladder distension, but this tends to be short-lived. Instillation therapy with dimethyl sulphoxide (DMSO), an industrial solvent, can help as the substance is thought to have a number of pharmacological actions, including local analgesia, anti-inflammatory activity and bacteriostasis. Treatment involves catheterization of the patient and instillation of 50 ml of 50% DMSO into the bladder. This is retained for 15–30 minutes before the

Table 10.1. *Systemic therapies for interstitial cystitis*

Drug	Mechanism
Antihistamines	Large numbers of mast cells present in bladders of women with interstitial cystitis. Histamine released may cause pain and inflammation
Heparin	Anti-inflammatory activity
Pentosan polysulphate	Augments the normal protective mucus layer of the bladder
Amitriptyline	Antidepressant with analgesic, anticholinergic and antihistaminic effects. Helps patient cope with symptoms

patient empties her bladder by voiding. Treatment is repeated every 1 or 2 weeks and up to six treatments may be necessary. A significant improvement can be expected in 50–80% of cases with early interstitial cystitis. Oxychlorosene can also be used in instillation therapy.

Surgical management of interstitial cystitis is frequently indicated and is generally undertaken in cases which fail to respond to conservative management. Procedures can be divided into endoscopic or open techniques. The former involves fulguration or resection of ulcers and is usually combined with other conservative therapies. Initial results with Nd:YAG laser therapy for this indication appear promising. Open surgery is used as a last resort and available options include partial cystectomy, augmentation cystoplasty, cystolysis and urinary diversion with or without cystectomy.

INCONTINENCE AND SEXUAL ACTIVITY

A number of women experience incontinence during sexual intercourse, possibly during penetration or during orgasm. Although the precise mechanism is unknown, it is thought to involve mechanical pressure or detrusor contraction. A change of position for intercourse may be beneficial, especially if mechanical pressure can be relieved. It is also helpful for the woman to empty her bladder as fully as possible before intercourse. Occasionally, therapy for a known bladder dysfunction, such as unstable detrusor, may cure the problem.

NOCTURNAL ENURESIS

On initial consultation, the true nature of the problem should be explained to the parents and the child and they should be reassured that the problem is a very common disorder and not a pathological entity;

most children become dry spontaneously. Treatment is divided into behaviour modification and pharmacological support. It should be noted that treatment is associated with a placebo effect of up to 68% and there is a spontaneous resolution rate of about 15% per year.

Behaviour modification

A number of options exist for behaviour modification (Table 10.2). Enuresis alarms are the most effective treatment for nocturnal enuresis and consist of a detector connected to the bed or within the pyjamas. Drawbacks include the failure to awaken the child, false alarms, alarm failure and waking the rest of the family. Full parental support is needed as treatment takes up to 4 months. Efficacy rates of about 75% have been reported and although there is a relapse rate of 20–40%, repeat treatment will often result in cure.

Bladder training consists of teaching the child to hold urine for progressively longer periods of time and has a low success rate (less than 20%). Dry bed training involves lifting the child out to pass urine during the night. This conditioning approach can give good results, but is time consuming and demanding on the parents. Psychotherapy is still used to treat enuresis, despite little evidence to support it. Studies show a cure rate of 10–20%, but this may be explained by a placebo effect. Responsibility reinforcement entails getting the child to take responsibility, e.g. star charts, rewards, punishments. Results tend to be mixed and depend very much on the individual child. Hypnotherapy appears to be successful, although time consuming, in the small trials that have been conducted.

> A number of options for behaviour modification can be applied, including alarms, bladder training and hypnotherapy.

Table 10.2. *Behaviour modification treatment for nocturnal enuresis*

- Enuresis alarms
- Bladder training
- Dry bed training
- Psychotherapy
- Responsibility reinforcement
- Hypnotherapy

Pharmacological treatment

A large number of drugs have been used to treat nocturnal enuresis, but only desmopressin and tricyclic antidepressants have been shown to benefit monosymptomatic nocturnal enuresis.

Desmopressin

Desmopressin (des amino-D-arginine vasopressin; DDAVP) is a synthetic analogue of vasopressin (ADH) and is currently the drug of choice for this problem. It acts on the ADH receptor to decrease urine production, but, unlike endogenous vasopressin, has little vasoactive affect. Desmopressin can be used in combination with behavioural measures.

Desmopressin is available as a nasal spray or tablets, both providing improvements in 75% of children and cure in 10–40%. Treatment should be stopped for evaluation after 3 months and other options considered if necessary. Unfortunately, relapse rates are high (> 70%) when treatment is discontinued. Desmopressin is well tolerated, and is safe for long term use.

Tricyclic antidepressants

Tricyclic antidepressants have a wide range of properties that may contribute to their therapeutic efficacy in enuresis, particularly their anticholinergic effects. Imipramine (Tofranil) is the most commonly prescribed agent of this type and has a similar success rate as desmopressin. However, it is associated with considerable side-effects (e.g. typical anticholinergic effects described in Chapter 8, hypotension and, rarely, cardiac rhythm disturbances). As with desmopressin, there is a high relapse rate when treatment is discontinued. Treatment with imipramine should not be for periods greater than 3 months without assessment.

Other drugs used with limited success include oxybutinin and non-steroidal anti-inflammatories.

A management strategy for the treatment of nocturnal enuresis is shown in Fig. 10.1.

> Only desmopressin and tricyclic antidepressants have been shown to benefit monosymptomatic nocturnal enuresis.

INCONTINENCE IN THE ELDERLY

General as well as specific therapeutic measures are of particular importance in the management of lower urinary tract dysfunction in the elderly. General measures that may be applied are shown in Table 10.3. It is impor-

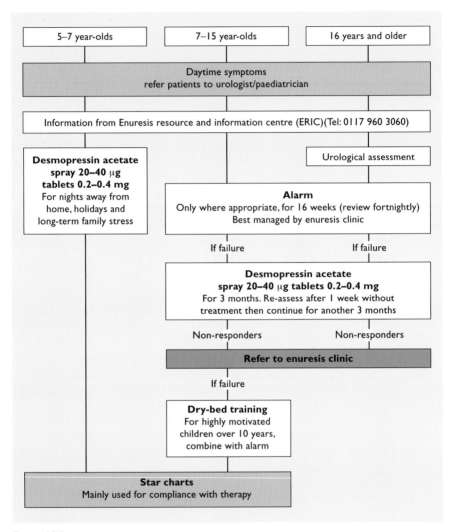

Figure 10.1.
A management strategy for the treatment of nocturnal enuresis (NHS Clinical Guidelines, UK., 1996).

tant to review drug therapy to ensure that all medications are appropriate and to minimize unwanted side-effects. This is particularly relevant for diuretic therapy, which can unnecessarily exacerbate urinary symptoms.

Regular toileting (e.g. 2-hour intervals) can improve incontinence considerably. Specific therapeutic measures include pelvic floor physiotherapy, bladder retraining, electrical stimulation therapy, drug therapy, surgery and catheterization. The decision on the most appropriate management regimen is often not easy and depends on a number of factors, including the complexity and severity of the bladder dysfunction, the mental and functional status of the patient, and the family and social support that is available.

General as well as specific therapeutic measures are of particular importance in the management of lower urinary tract dysfunction in the elderly.

Table 10.3. *General therapeutic measures for treating incontinence in the elderly*

- Treat any urinary tract infection
- Treat constipation
- Maximize mobility
- Improve toilet access
- Assess medications
- Rationalize fluid intake
- Ensure regular toileting

II PRACTICAL MANAGEMENT

Incontinence aids deal with the problem of incontinence, but as they do not cure it, they are not generally used in the first line of management. However, for some patients, such as the elderly and disabled, pads may be the only practical method of control. They can also be used as a temporary measure while objective investigation is undertaken or treatment awaited.

The range of products available, both on prescription and privately, is vast and often an inappropriate aid may be used. Before any incontinence aid can be prescribed or allocated, a full assessment of the patient's needs will be required to ensure optimal benefit. This is generally conducted in the patient's home by a district nurse or a continence advisor. The following points should be considered:

- Degree and type of incontinence
- Lifestyle of patient, e.g. employment, personal relationships, social activities
- Mobility and dexterity
- Toilet facilities
- Availability of carer
- Concurrent medication
- Fluid balance.

In the UK, pads are not prescribed on FP10. Generally, NHS Trusts provide disposable incontinence pads or reusable bed covers; the number of items is referred to as the daily allowance. The availability may vary across the country and this needs to be clarified by the local continence advisor. Other aids, such as catheters and leg bags, can be prescribed. Up-to-date information on products currently available with price guides can be found in The Continence Products Directory (The Continence Foundation, see Chapter 6).

Incontinence aids deal with the problem of incontinence, but they are not generally used in first-line management. Before any incontinence aid can be prescribed or allocated, a full assessment of the patient's needs will be required to ensure optimal benefit.

PADS

A vast array of pads made from various material exists, but their general purpose and properties are the same (Fig. 11.1). Materials used include wood pulp, with or without superabsorbent polymers. These polymers are capable of absorbing 50 times their own weight under some degree of pressure. Fluff (wood) pulps are cheaper, but only hold five times their weight beneath pressures typically found under a seated or supine person. Shape and the frequency of changing the pad are also important for performance. Pads can be designed for different purposes, ranging from light daytime urinary incontinence through to double incontinence.

> Pads can be designed for different purposes, ranging from light daytime urinary incontinence through to double incontinence.

Absorbent roll

Not used as frequently as shaped pads, absorbent roll is really only useful for light incontinence. It has the advantage, however, of being cut to suit an individual's requirements. Absorbent rolls are made from cellulose with cotton wool facing and a net cover. Pieces are used with stretch net or pouch pants or normal underwear.

Plastic-backed pads

This type of pad is used extensively and comes in various weights, shapes and sizes, as well as containing superabsorbers or not. They are generally fixed in place in the patients' own underwear or in mesh pants with a self-adhesive strip. One major disadvantage of these pads is that they can bulk up and, if not changed appropriately, the outside covering can come apart.

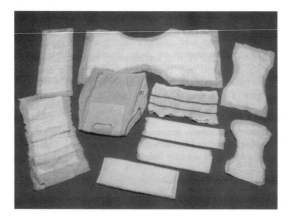

Figure 11.1.
Pads used for urinary incontinence.

Pouch pads
This type of pad is not plastic backed and is used with the marsupial or pouch pant system. The size of the pad depends on the pouch used and the degree of incontinence; they are frequently used in cases of light to moderate incontinence. This type of system is not very hygienic as urine passes through the pants (which are not changed) to get to the pad.

Washable pads
Some pads are reusable and are made of a special polyester with waterproof backing. They can be worn with normal underwear or stretch pants.

All-in-one pads
These are similar to babies nappies and are worn without additional pants. There additional side-fastening make them particularly suitable for disabled patients, and they can be used for heavy urinary incontinence.

PANTS

Numerous designs of pants are available which can be adapted to suit the severity and type of incontinence. Important factors to consider are mobility, possible spasticity of the limbs and manual dexterity. Pants should be fitted without being too tight and care should be taken to ensure the fabric does not damage the skin at the waist or the groin. Most products are reusable.

> Numerous designs of pants are available and important factors to consider are mobility, possible spasticity of the limbs and manual dexterity.

Stretch pants
Stretch pants are made from washable nylon net and are lightweight. They are used with varying sizes of plastic-backed pads.

Marsupial pants
Marsupial pants are made from a one-way fabric with a pouch into which a pad can be fitted (Fig. 11.2). They have the advantage of being able to change the pad without removing the garment. Pants with a plastic gusset should not be used with plastic-backed pads as a double layer of plastic will encourage skin irritation and chaffing. The disadvantage of this system is that the soiled garment remains in contact with skin, even when the pad is removed.

Waterproof pants
Waterproof pants look like babies plastic pants but are not recommended because of skin chafing, irritation and local infection.

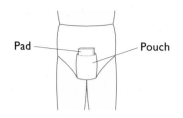

Figure 11.2.
Marsupial pants.

Washable pants

Washable pants have a special absorbent gusset that will soak up urine and can therefore be used without a pad. They are useful for light incontinence.

LEG BAGS

Leg bags are attached to a urethral or supra-pubic catheter and are designed to hold varying volumes of urine; capacities of 350 ml, 500 ml or 750 ml are available. Outlet taps vary to suit different types of manual dexterity. The bags can be attached to a waist belt or thigh or leg support straps; men tend to wear calf leg bags, while women wear thigh bags.

COLLECTING DEVICES

Collecting devices are essentially portable toilets. They are designed to fit over the vulva in women or the penis in men.

Female collecting devices

The female anatomy does not lend itself well to body-worn devices and it is hard to create a leak-proof seal. The appliances are also difficult to manage for less dextrous patients; however, they can be useful in wheelchair-bound patients. The devices are hand-held and can be placed over the vulva at a moment's notice. Examples include the Bridge urinal (Fig. 11.3), the St. Peter's boat, the Pantype female urinal and the swan-necked female urinal.

> Collecting devices are designed to fit over the vulva in women or the penis in men.

Male collecting devices

There is greater potential with the male anatomy for the successful use of collecting devices. Three types of male collecting devices are available: body-worn appliances, dribble pouches and penile sheaths.

Body-worn appliances

Body-worn appliances are held in position with waist and groin straps. Drip type urinals are designed for men with light to moderate incontinence. They consist of an internal sheath and an external cone in which urine is collected (Fig. 11.4). Pubic pressure urinals assist in penile retraction through the presence of a semi-rigid pubic pressure flange, which is held closely to the pubis and allows the penis to protrude into the urinal (Fig. 11.5). The penis passes through a flexible diaphragm into the urinal in the diaphragm urinal device, while penile and scrotal urinals are designed to contain the entire genitalia and can be used with a severely retracted penis.

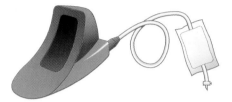

Figure 11.3.
The Bridge urinal.

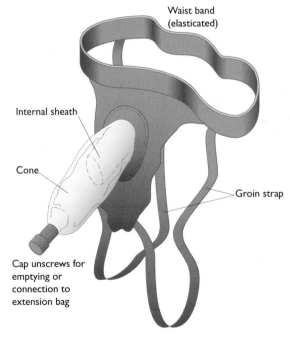

Waist band (elasticated)

Internal sheath

Cone

Groin strap

Cap unscrews for emptying or connection to extension bag

Figure 11.4.
Drip type urinal.

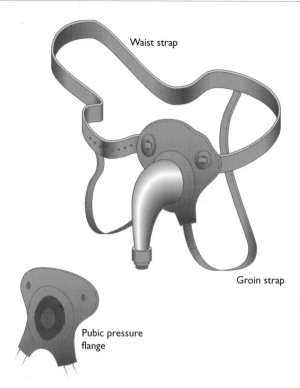

Waist strap

Groin strap

Pubic pressure
flange

Figure 11.5.
Pubic pressure urinal.

Dribble pouches

Dribble pouches are used in men with very slight or dribbling incontinence. They are made of waterproof backing with an absorbent pulp inner (Fig. 11.6). Newer versions contain superabsorbent material, making them less bulky and more discrete.

Penile sheaths

The penile sheath consists of a soft latex sleeve that fits over the penis and connects to a urine collection bag (Fig. 11.7). Other descriptive terms for this device are incontinence sheath, condom urinal or external male catheter. This type of urine collection system is suitable for men with moderate to severe urinary incontinence and for those with urgency or frequency. Different types of sheaths are available, but generally the thicker, less flexible latex version with anti-kink moulding is most successful. Nonlatex sheaths have been developed to help men with skin sensitivity. A reasonable degree of manual dexterity, vision and mental ability are required to use this appliance.

Penis inserted in pouch

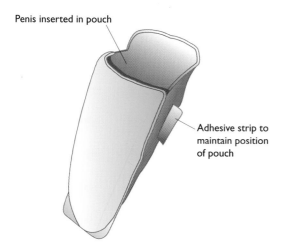

Figure 11.6.
Male dribble pouch.

Adhesive strip to
maintain position
of pouch

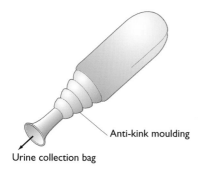

Figure 11.7.
Penile sheaths.

Anti-kink moulding

Urine collection bag

12 MISCONCEPTIONS AND FREQUENTLY ASKED QUESTIONS

There are many commonly held misconceptions concerning urinary incontinence. The following statements and questions have been made repeatedly, by both patients and professionals. By stating established facts, areas of misunderstanding can be clarified, and this will help to improve education and allay anxiety.

Urinary incontinence is normal
Involuntary loss of urine is never normal. In certain situations, it may be short-lived (e.g. during or immediately following pregnancy) or self-limiting. However, persistent symptoms indicate pathology and warrant investigation and appropriate treatment.

Nothing can be done to overcome my incontinence
On the contrary, most cases of urinary incontinence may be cured or significantly improved, once the cause has been established. Advice on simple measures to alleviate symptoms is available from general practitioners, district nurses and continence advisors. However, referral at an early stage for urodynamic investigation may reduce treatment failures and disillusionment among patients.

Why did my incontinence start after I had a baby?
This is a very common claim which is often difficult to verify. Many women experience urinary symptoms for the first time during pregnancy, and these may persist following the birth of the baby. This may be perceived by the mother as a direct result of delivery rather than of the pregnancy as a whole. Urinary incontinence may arise directly as a result of pudendal nerve and pelvic floor damage following labour, but evidence suggests that a proportion of women develop detrusor instability during pregnancy which may persist following delivery. If urinary incontinence persists after the puerperium, then urodynamic investigation is indicated.

Incontinence runs in my family

Apart from rare forms of muscular dystrophy, which may give rise to GSI, there is no simple genetic basis for urinary incontinence. However, a familial element may be present, especially in the case of detrusor instability and nocturnal enuresis. This is often the result of abnormal `potty training', carried out by a parent with the condition, which leads to a reinforcement of abnormal behaviour patterns resulting in urinary symptoms.

Drinking plenty will help my bladder problems

Unless symptoms are secondary to a urinary tract infection, increased fluid intake will only exacerbate symptoms of frequency, urgency and incontinence. Excessive intake should be discouraged, but drastic reduction should also be avoided, especially in the elderly. The usual recommendation is 1–1.5 litres per day.

Will I have to take these tablets forever?

The treatment of detrusor instability is primarily pharmacological, using anticholinergic agents. Such drugs do not affect the underlying pathological process (often unknown), but merely provide symptomatic relief. Symptoms usually return on cessation of treatment. It is common, however, to note spontaneous waxing and waning of the symptoms of detrusor instability, and therefore drug therapy may be reduced in times of remission. Because the therapeutic effect of most anticholinergic agents is paralleled by their side-effects, patients should be encouraged to alter the dose of their medication to suit their needs. A dose reduction may be tried when side-effects are troublesome, or when at home and in easy reach of the toilet. Conversely, increased dosage should be recommended to provide maximum cover, e.g. when out shopping or socializing. For oxybutinin this can be achieved relatively easily as it is a drug with a short half-life.

I've tried pelvic floor exercises, but they didn't help me

Many women believe that their symptoms are due to weak pelvic floor muscles following childbirth. For women with detrusor instability this assumption is not valid, and pelvic floor exercises are of little benefit. Pelvic floor contractions are commonly taught to women following delivery, or when they complain of urinary incontinence. The belief is that pelvic floor training may prevent or even cure urinary incontinence. These exercises are usually carried out without supervision or vaginal examination, for example in an aerobics class, and are often incorrectly performed. There is little evidence to suggest that performing postnatal exercises protects against future incontinence. Even supervised Kegel exercises in women with proven GSI result in few complete cures. Most women will, however, derive a degree of symptomatic relief, and should be taught pelvic floor contractions properly, with clear knowledge of their limitations.

I don't want to end up smelling of urine when I'm old

Urinary incontinence conjures up the image of an elderly person surrounded by an ammoniacal odour. Even if the underlying problem cannot be cured, modern incontinence aids and appliances are available to help contain urinary leakage. Soiling of clothes should not occur with appropriate pads or pants. Correct medical and nursing management should ensure that the distress caused by urinary incontinence in the elderly is alleviated. Many women use sanitary towels, which are unsuitable and cause skin excoriation. Modern incontinence pads are expensive, but can usually be provided free to people in the community, who should contact their local continence advisor for information.

Is post-micturition dribble a sign of prostate disease?

No, this symptom is much more likely to be related to loss of perineal muscle tone with pooling in the bulbar urethra. The patient can be taught to massage the remaining urine out after micturition (see Chapter 3).

Can constipation cause retention and incontinence?

In the elderly, particularly when there is associated cerebrovascular disease, incontinence can occur secondary to a high residual urine and faecal impaction. With attention to the bowel, intermittent self-catheterization on a temporary basis until bladder control is achieved will often resolve the problem.

Can incontinence be cured in the confused elderly?

The use of a bladder diary to look for a pattern will help, as well as observing typical gestures, body language and checking the relationship between eating and toileting. This will allow a management plan to be developed which can offer a high success rate.

What do I do when a male patient is determined not to have a catheter, despite regular incontinence due to obstruction?

Counsel the patient and offer a choice of a sheath system and or a pubic pressure appliance once the obstruction has been eliminated.

Are antiseptic bladder installations useful?

Published evidence suggests only a limited role for antiseptic bladder installations in the management of catheterized patients and there is little evidence that their use is associated with reduced rates of urinary tract infection.

If I break a closed or linked drainage system to administer an installation, do I need to change the leg bag?

Any breakage of a closed or linked drainage system will inevitably introduce contamination and therefore the leg bag should be changed on every occasion.

In patients with indwelling catheters, should regular cleaning of the urethral meatus take place?

Regular cleaning of the urethral meatus may cause urethritis and this may increase susceptibility to urine tract infection. The urothelial cells are fragile and shedding has been demonstrated, even when physiological saline is used as a mechanical irrigant. However, the area should be washed and dried daily and skin condition checked.

Why don't patients who develop bacteriuria during long-term catheterization develop systemic symptoms?

Approximately 90% of all long-term catheterized patients developed bacteriuria within a week of initial insertion. This is partly due to loss of the flushing action of urine which allows infection between the external catheter surface and the urethral tissue. Some protection from the systemic invasion may be due to the mucus layer on the bladder surface which protects against tissue invasion.

How do I treat over-granulation and bleeding at the insertion site of a supra-pubic catheter?

The granulation tissue should be treated by cauterization with a silver nitrate tip.

Are disposable single use catheters less likely to cause problems in patients requiring intermittent self-catheterization?

Re-usable catheters are much less expensive than the single use products. On the whole, single use products should be reserved for patients with neuropathic bladder disorders who are at high risk of infection and for patients with urethral strictures or recurrent urinary tract infections. Indeed, research suggests that unlubricated catheters causes stricture formation.

The patient's catheter blocks every 3 days, what should I do?

Upon removal of a catheter check that the eyelets are actually blocked and that the catheter is not bypassing as above. If the eyelets are blocked:

- Change the type of catheter to 100% silicone, as the lumen of these catheters are larger and silicone, being totally inert, attracts less crystallization
- Encourage the patient to drink – suggest two glasses of cranberry juice per day
- Vitamin C, 4 g/day, has been found to be beneficial if the patient can tolerate it.

If I do not know what size catheter a patient uses and I am unable to specify the size on the prescription what size will be dispensed? Does increasing the size help to stop leakage?

The drug tariff in the UK instructs that size 14 or 16 should be supplied if no size is specified on the prescription. A size 12 female length should be used in women unless they are particularly large and a size 14–16 standard length in men. Increasing the size of the catheter in cases of leakage is a common mistake. Larger catheters (16 and above) are more likely to cause bypassing of urine around the catheter than the smaller sizes due to the higher pressure exerted on the urethral wall. To avoid bypassing, use the smallest size of catheter you can get away with to provide adequate drainage. Larger sizes are also more likely to cause urethral strictures.

Why should I only use sterile water when inflating a catheter balloon?

Water is the only acceptable fluid as normal saline will crystallize and block the inflation tube. This makes catheter removal very difficult and may need hospital admission. Importantly, never cut off the inflation valve.

How many people are affected by incontinence?

Approximately 5% of the UK population (about three million people) are affected by incontinence, and this figure is rising with our ageing population. However, it is not solely a problem for the elderly. Incontinence is particularly prevalent among, for example, women aged between 20 and 50 years, but early treatment reduces the long-term cost of later continence treatment.

What percentage of 5-year-old children are enuretic?

Approximately 15% of this age group are still having problems and approximately 16% of these remit each year.

What severity of enuresis warrants intervention?

During a 2-week period, 50% or more wet nights is considered a significant problem. Organize a diary and keep a record of wetting for at least 4 weeks, i.e. the number of wet nights per week, the wetting time and the size of the patch.

Who are Continence Advisors and what can a Continence Advisor offer?

Continence Advisors are fully qualified nurses who have undergone specialist training in the field of incontinence. They can offer a range of help, including:

- An in depth assessment of the patient's incontinence problem, often with aid of diagnostic equipment, e.g. bladder scanner, flow meter, perineometry
- Programmes of treatment to help the sufferer regain continence
- Advice to patients, carers and relatives on how to manage the continence problem in their own home
- Advice and information on the provision of continence aids and appliances.

Now my stress incontinence is cured do I still need to continue with the pelvic floor exercises?

Yes, pelvic floor exercises are for life and should be continued on a continuing regimen.

Where can I get pads and pants?

Most NHS Trusts or Health Districts have a home delivery service for pads and pants. However, this is often restricted due to financial restraints, i.e. waiting lists and rationing of type and amount allocated to each patient. No incontinence products will be issued without a full continence assessment by a trained nurse.

Can my continence problem be made worse by what I eat and drink?

Yes, there is a long list of foods and beverages that can contribute to a bladder instability problem including:

- Alcoholic and carbonated drinks
- Soft drinks containing caffeine
- Tomato-based products
- Tea and coffee (even decaffeinated coffee can cause bladder irritation to a certain extent)
- Citrus juices and whole fruits
- Highly seasoned or spicy foods
- Sugar including honey
- Artificial sweeteners.

It is worth keeping a diary of food and drink along with bladder pattern.

As a man, I do not wish to use a female pad to manage my incontinence. What else is available?

There are male incontinence pads now available, but many men prefer to use other continence devices. The sheath and drainage bag system is useful if the patient has a penile length of at least 2.5 cm. If the patient has a retracted penis, then a pubic pressure appliance may be more suitable. All of these devices are available on prescription.

I have been offered electrical stimulation for my incontinence, how does this work?

Electrical stimulation aims to restore muscle tone and strengthen and help normalize muscle function. It can promote continence by improving pelvic floor tone and increasing patients awareness of their pelvic floor muscles. In addition, an overactive detrusor muscle can be suppressed by electrical stimulation.

INDEX